PASS PARAMEDIC!

Bruce R. Shade, EMT-P
Commissioner of EMS
City of Cleveland
President, NAEMT

Publisher: David T. Culverwell
Editor: Claire Merrick
Assistant Editor: Lisa Esposito
Project Manager: Patricia Stinecipher

1st Edition

Printed in the United States of America

Mosby–Year Book, Inc.
11830 Westline Industrial Drive
St. Louis, Missouri 63146

ISBN 0-8151-0040-X

Preface

Each day, paramedics throughout the country provide emergency care to hundreds of thousands of persons experiencing medical and traumatic emergencies. Staying current is an important part of ensuring that the best care is provided at all times to all patients.

The National Registry of EMTs is the nationally recognized agency for certifying paramedics and documenting their level of competence according to the recommended standard of care. The primary goal of National Registry certification is to ensure that each paramedic possesses the knowledge and skills necessary to manage patients through various medical and traumatic emergencies. Since the inception of National Registry certification, thousands of health care providers have successfully completed the exam process. Today, these health care providers are delivering quality care to millions of patients.

This pocket-sized booklet is designed to be carried with you while preparing for the National Registry exam or your state certification exam or practicing in the clinical setting. It includes all the essential information you need to function according to the 1985 D.O.T. paramedic curriculum and the 1992 ACLS guidelines.

Contents

Section 1

Using this guide
How the National Registry and state certification exams are conducted
Avoiding test-related anxiety

Using This Guide

This pocket-sized guide is designed to be carried with you while preparing for the National Registry or your state certification exam. It contains all the essential information needed to successfully complete the practical skills portion of the exam. It is also a useful tool that can be carried with you when functioning in the clinical setting.

Section 1 of this guide focuses on:

- how the National Registry/state exams are conducted and required testing stations.
- hints for dealing with exam-related anxiety.

Section 2 of this guide includes:

- skill station testing information.
- skill step listings and helpful hints for each of the primary skills.

Section 3 of this guide includes:

- concise information on ECG dysrhythmias including key characteristics.

Section 4 of this guide includes:

- step-by-step ACLS treatment algorithms.

Section 5 of this guide includes:

- concise information on the primary cardiac medications.

This guide keeps in mind the difficulty of being a National Registry or state certification candidate and/or functioning paramedic. Its compact and flip-open design allows you to place it next to you no matter where you are or what you are doing. To get the greatest benefit, carry this guide in your pocket so that you can refer to it in times of need. This includes while waiting to practice skills in the various stations. **The more you review, the more you learn.**

How National Registry/State Certification Exams Are Conducted

The typical National Registry exam or state certification exam lasts one day. Usually, during the first portion of the day you take the written examination. To prepare for the written exam you should study your paramedic textbook paying special attention to assuring your comprehension of the D.O.T. learning objectives. It is said that if you know the D.O.T. learning objectives you will pass most written exams. The latter part of the day is then directed to testing your ability to perform the following skills:

- Patient assessment and management
- Airway adjuncts, bag-valve-mask, and endotracheal intubation
- Intravenous cannulation, IV bolus, and piggyback medication administration
- Static and dynamic ECG dysrhythmia recognition including treatments and electrical therapy
- Spinal immobilization (seated patient)
- Random basic skills
    - Spinal Immobilization (Lying Patient)
    - Bleeding-Wounds-Shock
    - Long Bone Splinting
    - Traction Splinting

Avoiding Examination Anxiety

Much of the anxiety associated with participating in the National Registry or state certification exam can be alleviated through proper preexamination preparation. To further reduce tension, learn the appropriate "station etiquette." This means there are certain behaviors you can display which enhance your chances of passing. First, understand that the evaluators are there to evaluate your proficiency with the advanced and basic skills outlined in this guide. Treat them with the appropriate respect and courtesy. Understand that when they document your performance, it is in an effort to make sure you have achieved the appropriate standards. Don't assume that you are the only one who is nervous as it may be the first time some of the evaluators have tested candidates. Also, most evaluators share something in common with you, the experience of being a student at one point or another. Employ the following while in the testing stations:

- Display an appropriate sense of confidence. This conveys to the instructor that you know what you are doing. However, be careful not to come off as being "cocky."
- Make a habit of verbalizing the skill steps in addition to actually performing them. This communicates to the evaluator(s) through two mediums and assures that the evaluator sees or hears you perform each step.

Section 2

Skill station testing information
Skill listings

Special Information

- Depending on your local instruction or protocols, it may be acceptable to do steps earlier or later in the skill. These are noted by the * symbol.
- In the testing stations it is acceptable to verbalize some actions. These are represented by the ☺ symbol.
- Also, you should ask the evaluator, "What do I find?" or "Do I find anything abnormal?" where you see the ⌧ symbol.
- The ✓ symbol means that you should check something.
- **Bolded** points are considered critical tasks that **must** be performed.

Skill Station Testing Information

1. PATIENT ASSESSMENT/MANAGEMENT

Upon entering the patient assessment testing area there is typically an instructor standing in front of a moulaged victim who is lying on the floor. The simulated victim is used to test your assessment skills and ability to manage a multi-system trauma victim. You are required to perform a "hands-on," head-to-toe, physical assessment and voice treatment of a moulaged victim for a given scenario. This station includes:

- Primary Survey/Resuscitation
- Secondary Survey

2. VENTILATORY MANAGEMENT

Upon entering the airway testing area there is typically an instructor standing or sitting in front of a table where an intubation manikin and airway management equipment are placed. Given a scenario of having just found an apneic patient with a palpable pulse, you must demonstrate immediate, aggressive management of the patient using simple airway adjuncts, bag-valve-mask device, supplemental oxygen, and successful placement of an endotracheal tube (ET).

3. CARDIAC ARREST SKILLS

The candidate's ability to manage cardiac arrests and interpret ECGs is verified in two portions:

- Dynamic Cardiology
- Static Cardiology

Upon entering the cardiac arrest testing area there is typically an instructor standing or sitting in front of a table where a defibrillator manikin and defibrillator are placed. You are evaluated in your ability to manage codes, including actual delivery of electrical therapy, and "voicing" all interpretations and other treatments given a scenario. The presentation of this portion is similar to the American Heart Association's "megacode."

In the second portion of the testing station you are given four (4) prepared ECG tracings with associated vital patient information. You must verbalize the interpretation of the dysrhythmia and all associated treatments. A sample case is presented on page 56.

4. IV AND MEDICATION SKILLS

This station consists of three interrelated parts:

- Intravenous Therapy
- Intravenous Bolus Medications
- Intravenous Piggyback Medications

Upon entering the IV and medication testing station there is typically an instructor standing or sitting in front of a table where an IV arm, IV equipment/solutions and various medications are placed. You are required to establish a patent IV in the manikin arm, administer an IV bolus of medication and then mix, hang, and administer an IV piggyback drip of medication appropriate for the given scenario.

5. SPINAL IMMOBILIZATION (SEATED PATIENT)

Using any type of half-spine immobilization device (wooden board, commercial vest-type), you must demonstrate appropriate application and spinal immobilization.

6. RANDOM BASIC SKILLS

You need to demonstrate acceptable performance of two (2) of the following skills tested at random:

- Spinal Immobilization (Lying Patient)
- Bleeding-Wounds-Shock
- Long Bone Splinting
- Traction Splinting

Patient Assessment/Management

1. **Employ infection control procedures.** ☺

Airway with C-Spine Control

2. **Provide (or direct your partners) manual in-line immobilization of patient's head.**
3. Say to patient, "Are you OK? Can you hear me? I am here to help you."
4. **Open and assess the airway, using the modified jaw thrust.** ⌦
   - *if snoring heard or patient unconscious:* insert an oral or nasopharyngeal airway or perform endotracheal intubation using neutral in-line immobilization technique.
   - *if gurgling heard or secretions/blood/vomitus present:* suction the upper airway.

Breathing

5. ✓ **breathing.** ⌦
   - quickly inspect neck for jugular vein distention, tracheal shift, or tugging.
   - listen for breathing and look for adequacy of chest rise.
   - inspect chest for deformities, holes, or bruising.
   - palpate chest for equal expansion (symmetry).
   - auscultate lung sounds.
6. **Initiate oxygen therapy.** ☺
   - 100% via nonrebreather mask, bag-valve-mask, or demand valve device.
7. **Assure adequate ventilation of patient.** ☺
   - if breathing shallow, rapid (>20 breaths per minute), or slow (<10 breaths per minute) assist breathing with bag-valve-mask supplied with 10-15 liters of oxygen and a reservoir.
8. **Manage any injury that may compromise breathing.** ☺

- *open pneumothorax:* cover with an occlusive dressing, tape three sides down.
- *tension pneumothorax:* lift one side of the occlusive dressing, perform emergency chest decompression (insert 14-16 g. over-the-needle IV catheter with flutter valve attached, into 2nd intercostal space, at the midclavicular line).
- *flail chest:* immobilize with a bulky dressing or towels taped to the chest.

Circulation

9. **✓ for a pulse**. ⌦
   - radial (if present, indicates a B/P of at least 80 systolic).
   - femoral (if present, indicates B/P of at least 70 systolic).
   - carotid (if present, indicates B/P of at least 60 systolic).
10. **✓ peripheral perfusion**. ⌦
    - ✓ skin color, temperature, and capillary refill.
11. **Look for and control major bleeding.** ☺ ⌦
12. Take vital signs. ⌦
    - ✓ to see if patient's condition has changed; airway, breathing, and circulation.
    - ✓ BP (palpate the arm before applying cuff to make sure no injury is present).
13. **Apply or consider application of the pneumatic anti-shock garment (PASG).**
    - do secondary exam of body parts to be enclosed prior to application of garment.
14. **Initiate volume replacement** (usually deferred until the patient is loaded into the ambulance). ☺
    - initiate two large-bore IV lines.
    - select appropriate IV solutions and administration sets (use Ringer's or normal saline and macrodrips if volume replacement needed).

Disability

15. Perform mini-neuro assessment: AVPU.* ⌧
16. **Apply a cervical collar**.* ☺
17. **Secure patient to full backboard** (may do this at same time as applying PASG).* ☺
18. **If indicated, call for immediate transport of the patient**.

Secondary Survey

19. Examine the head. ⌧
    - **✓ to see if patient's condition has changed (airway, breathing, circulation)**.
    - inspect mouth,* nose,* and assess facial area.
    - inspect and palpate scalp and ears.
    - ✓ eyes: PEARRL.
20. Examine the neck.* ⌧
    - ✓ position of trachea and jugular veins.
    - palpate the cervical spine.
21. Examine the chest.* ⌧
    - inspect for holes, deformity, or bruising.
    - palpate for symmetry.
    - auscultate lung sounds.
22. Examine the abdomen/pelvis.* ⌧
    - inspect and palpate abdomen.
    - palpate pelvis.
23. Examine the lower extremities.* ⌧
    - inspect and palpate left leg.

- inspect and palpate right leg.
- ✓ motor, sensory, and distal circulation in both legs.

24. Examine the upper extremities.* ⌦
    - inspect and palpate left arm.
    - inspect and palpate right arm.
    - ✓ motor, sensory, and distal circulation in both arms.
25. Examine the posterior thorax/lumbar and buttocks.* ⌦
    - inspect and palpate posterior thorax.
    - inspect and palpate lumbar and buttocks area.
26. Identify and treat minor wounds/fractures appropriately.
27. **✓ to see if patient's condition has changed (airway, breathing, circulation).**

Helpful Hints be sure to:

- ❑ **immediately establish and maintain spinal protection.**
- ❑ ✓ the ABCDs **FIRST** (airway, *then* breathing, *then* circulation, *then* disability), **appropriately managing any life-threatening conditions** along the way. You can vary this slightly by asking the patient if he or she can hear you as you open his or her airway. This gives you a sense of the patient's mental status (disability).
- ❑ in the testing situation continually ask the evaluator "How is the patient's airway, breathing, circulation, and disability? Has anything changed?" Then ask if you find anything after you evaluate each body area.
- ❑ examine back surface of patient's body when you are log-rolling him or her onto long backboard or PASG.
- ❑ **call for patient transport within 10 minutes, differentiate between "load & go" vs. "stay & treat."**
- ❑ **do your secondary exam AFTER you are en route to the trauma center.**

Endotracheal Intubation

To complete the skill, do the following:

1. **Employ infection control procedures.** ☹
2. Open the airway manually using the head-tilt/chin-lift or jaw thrust.
3. Place an oropharyngeal airway (or nasopharyngeal airway).
   - elevate tongue by grasping the jaw and tongue between the thumb and index finger of your left hand, and lift it anteriorly.
   - insert airway in a backward position along the roof of the mouth, and as the tip of the airway approaches the back of the throat near the base of the tongue, rotate airway 180° into its proper position (flange should rest on patient's lips).
4. **Assist the patient's breathing or ventilate with a bag-valve-mask**.
   - place mask on the patient's face with the narrow end (apex) over the bridge of the nose and wide end (base) in the groove between the lower lip and chin.
   - position one hand over the mask with your thumb on the dome, the index and middle fingers on the base, and the ring and little fingers under the patient's jaw.
   - press downward on mask to maintain an effective seal between patient's face and mask.
   - use your fingers to tilt patient's head back, and displace jaw forward.
   - squeeze bag as completely as possible to deliver sufficient ventilation to patient, watching the patient's chest rise during ventilation and collapse during passive exhalation.

- **connect a reservoir and oxygen tubing to the oxygen inlet of the bag-valve-mask and deliver oxygen at 12 to 15 liters per minute.**
- **ventilate the patient (12 to 20 times per minute with at least 800 ml of air).**
- auscultate chest to be sure adequate ventilation is being delivered. ⌦

5. **Ask your partner to hyperventilate the patient while you prepare your equipment.**
6. Select proper equipment for intubation and ✓ it.
   - connect laryngoscope blade to handle, ✓ light for brightness and tightness.
   - inflate and deflate distal cuff of ET tube to ✓ for leaks. Insert a stylette if desired. **Do not allow stylette to extend beyond the distal end of the tube.**
7. Remove oropharyngeal airway and place patient's head into a "sniffing" position.
8. Hold laryngoscope in your left hand.
9. Insert laryngoscope blade into right side of patient's mouth and sweep the tongue to the left.
10. Advance blade to the level of the vallecula (or over the epiglottis).
11. Visualize epiglottis, then gently lift laryngoscope handle at a 45° angle to the floor. **Do not use teeth as a fulcrum.**
12. Insert endotracheal (ET) tube into right side of patient's mouth and pass it between the vocal cords. Hold ET tube at its midpoint during insertion to give you more control over the direction of the tube.
13. Advance distal cuff of ET tube 1 to 2 cm past the vocal cords.
14. Inflate distal cuff of ET tube with enough air to occlude the airway **and disconnect syringe.**
15. Hold ET tube with one hand at all times to prevent accidental displacement.
16. Connect bag-valve-mask to ET tube, ✓ **for proper placement by watching for chest rise while delivering a ventilation with a bag-valve device.**

17. Recheck for proper placement.
    - visualize equal chest rise with each ventilation.
    - **auscultate the chest bilaterally and over the epigastrium (stomach) with a stethoscope.** ⌦
18. Direct your partner to take over ventilations.
19. Secure ET tube in place with tape, a tie, or a commercial device. ☺

Helpful Hints <u>be sure to</u>:

- ❑ **begin ventilations within 30 seconds after employing infection control procedures and avoid interruptions in ventilation of greater than 30 seconds at any time.** If an attempt is unsuccessful within 30 seconds, discontinue attempt, hyperventilate patient for at least 30 seconds, and reattempt intubation.
- ❑ test your equipment including patency of the distal ET tube cuff.
- ❑ place patient's head into a "sniffing" position before performing endotracheal intubation.
- ❑ limit each attempt (**maximum of three tries allowed in testing situation**) to **no more than 30 seconds**.
- ❑ avoid a fulcrum action as you lift the mandible with the laryngoscope. In other words, **stay off the teeth**.
- ❑ hold the ET tube at its midpoint during insertion to give you more control over the direction of the tube as it passes into the pharynx and trachea.
- ❑ **✓ for chest rise and auscultate lung sounds both before and after inflation of the distal cuff.**
- ❑ if tube is inserted too far (into mainstem bronchus) deflate distal cuff, withdraw tube slightly, reinflate cuff, and auscultate lung sounds to assure proper placement.

To complete this skill, do the following:

1. Employ infection control procedures. ☺
2. Determine the patient's status.
    - ✓ responsiveness/airway.
    - ✓ breathing.
    - ✓ pulse.
3. **Initiate CPR if indicated**. ☺
4. Assign team members. ☺
    - person to maintain airway and provide ventilations.
    - person to perform chest compressions.
    - person to establish an IV, administer medications, and document treatments given.
5. If the patient is unconscious bare patient's chest and perform "Quick Look" with the defibrillator paddles. If the patient is conscious attach the ECG leads.
6. Announce the name of the ECG dysrhythmia you see on the ECG monitor (see ECG dysrhythmias, starting on page 35).
7. **Direct the appropriate treatments** (see treatment algorithms, starting on page 57). Remember:
    - **treat the patient, not the ECG monitor**.
    - **order high concentrations of supplemental oxygen**.

If the patient is in cardiac arrest:

- defibrillation (skill steps listed on page 18) is the definitive treatment for ventricular fibrillation (VF) and pulseless ventricular tachycardia (VT), **deliver the initial shocks at the earliest possible time. Following the first three successive shocks, it is pretty much drug . . . shock . . . drug . . . shock**.
- **endotracheal intubation** and placing an IV lifeline (Ringer's or normal saline in the antecubital fossa) are done early in the management of cardiac arrest, typically preceding epinephrine administration.
- **epinephrine, 1 mg, is administered in all types of cardiac arrest (repeat q. 3-5 min)**.
- immediate transcutaneous pacing should be considered in the early management of asystole.
- **atropine, 1 mg, is administered in asystole, PEA, and bradycardia with hypotension** (repeat q. 3-5 min).
- **apply different interventions whenever appropriate indications exist**.

If the patient has a pulse:

- **synchronized cardioversion at 100 J, 200 J, 300 J, 360 J** (premedicate whenever possible) is administered in PSVT, atrial fibrillation/flutter, or ventricular tachycardia (with serious signs or symptoms). PSVT and atrial fibrillation/flutter may respond to lower energy levels, so start with 50 J.
- **vagal maneuver, and/or adenosine at 6 mg, rapid IV push (1-3 seconds) repeated at 12 mg in 1-2 minutes, are administered in PSVT** (without serious signs or symptoms).
- **lidocaine, 1-1.5 mg/kg, IV push (repeated at 0.5-0.75 mg/kg, IV push, q. 5-10 min. to a total of 3 mg/kg) is administered in wide-complex tachycardia of unknown origin or ventricular tachycardia** (without serious signs or symptoms).

8. Look for a change in rhythm.

9. ✓ the patient's pulse, and if appropriate his or her respirations and BP.
10. **Interpret and manage next rhythm.**
    - **lidocaine, 1.5 mg/kg, is administered in VF/pulseless VT (repeat q. 3-5 min. to a total loading dose of 3 mg/kg) following the first series of defibrillation (200 J, 200-300 J, 360 J), epinephrine administration and the fourth defibrillation.**
    - **defibrillation at 360 joules follows lidocaine administration in VF/pulseless VT.**
11. Look for a change in rhythm.
12. ✓ the patient's pulse, and if appropriate the respirations and BP.
13. **Interpret and manage next rhythm**. If rhythm is restored but it is a slow rhythm with hypotension treat with:
    - **atropine, 0.5 to 1 mg, IV push. Repeat as needed up to a total of 0.04 mg/kg.**
    - **in refractory bradycardia, initiate transcutaneous pacing, or administer dopamine, 5 to 20 mcg/kg/minute, IV infusion.**
14. Look for a change in rhythm.
15. ✓ the patient's pulse and, if appropriate his or her respirations and BP.
16. **Interpret and manage the next rhythm**. If defibrillation restores an effective electromechanical rhythm with a normal rate or tachycardia and the blood pressure is adequate treat the patient with:
    - **prophylactic lidocaine, 1-1.5 mg/kg, IV push followed by a lidocaine infusion of 2-4 mg/min.**

Helpful Hints be sure to:

❑ **deliver prompt defibrillation in the management of VF/pulseless VT.**
❑ administer epinephrine in all types of cardiac arrest.

Defibrillation (indicated if VF/pulseless VT is present)

To complete this skill, do the following:

1. Prepare equipment, apply conductive gel to paddles or place prepackaged gel pads on patient's chest.
2. Charge defibrillator to 200 J and apply paddles to patient's chest using 20-25 pounds of pressure.
    - place one paddle to the right of the upper sternum just below the right clavicle.
    - place one paddle laterally in the left midclavicular line.
3. Re-verify ECG rhythm before defibrillating.
4. **Loudly instruct everyone to "stand back" while clearing yourself from contact with patient or anything touching patient**.
5. **Simultaneously press the buttons on both defibrillator paddles to deliver shock**.
6. ✓ rhythm after delivering shock. Verbalize your findings.
7. If rhythm is still VF/pulseless VT, **immediately recharge defibrillator and perform a second defibrillation at 200-300 J**. ✓ rhythm after shock has been delivered. Verbalize your findings.
8. If patient remains in VF/pulseless VT, **immediately recharge defibrillator and deliver a third successive shock at 360 J. As needed, subsequent defibrillations are delivered at 360 J. ✓ pulse before and after each subsequent shock.**
9. **If patient remains pulseless, remove paddles and direct CPR to be continued**.

Helpful Hints be sure to:

- ❑ **deliver first shock in a timely manner, without delay other than to do CPR with simple adjuncts.**
- ❑ **deliver second/third shocks without delay other than time required to reassess and recharge paddles.**

Intravenous Therapy

<u>To complete this skill, do the following</u>:

1. Check selected IV fluid to make sure it is:
    - the proper solution (*typically* Ringer's, or normal saline are used for trauma and cardiac arrest, D_5W for medical).
    - clear.
    - not outdated.
    - not leaking.
2. Select appropriate catheter (14-16 g. for trauma, 18-20 g. for medical).
3. Select proper administration set (macro for trauma, micro for medical and drug administration).
4. Prepare IV bag and administration set.
    - remove IV bag from its protective envelope and protective cap from administration set.
    - invert IV bag.
    - using sterile techniques, insert spiked end of administration set into fluid port of IV bag.
    - close off flow control valve, turn IV bag right side up, and squeeze drip chamber two or three times to fill it half way.
    - open control valve to flush tubing (to remove any air).
5. Cut or tear several lengths of tape.*
6. **Exercise infection control precautions.** ☺
7. Place patient into suitable position with selected extremity lower than heart.

8. Apply tourniquet and palpate suitable vein.
9. **Cleanse site appropriately**.
10. Perform venipuncture **without contaminating equipment or site**.
    - hold needle at a 45° angle to skin.
    - penetrate skin with bevel of needle pointed up.
    - enter vein with needle, and advance it until tip of catheter is well within the vein.
    - note when blood fills flashback chamber of needle. ☺
    - occlude vein proximal to catheter with your little finger to prevent blood loss.
    - while holding catheter stable, remove needle (stylette).
    - connect IV tubing to catheter.
11. Release tourniquet.*
12. Open IV flow control valve and run IV for a brief period of time to assure line is patent.
13. Secure catheter in place with tape or a commercial device.
14. Adjust flow rate as appropriate for case.
15. **Dispose of needle in proper biomedical waste container**. ☺

Helpful Hints be sure to:

- ❑ check the IV fluid before its use.
- ❑ release the tourniquet once the IV tubing is connected to the cannula.
- ❑ continually employ infection control procedures.
- ❑ discard the needle appropriately.

- ❑ **in the testing station, your limit for establishing a patent and properly adjusted IV is up to three attempts over 6 minutes.**
- ❑ **not contaminate the IV equipment or site. If you do you must correct the situation before proceeding.**
- ❑ **avoid any improper technique that will result in the potential for catheter shear or air embolism.**

Additional Considerations

- lactated Ringer's or normal saline is used in the management of cardiac arrest. The IV should be placed in the antecubital fossa.
- use the formula below to calculate IV solution drip rates per minute:

$$\text{gtt/min} = \frac{\text{volume to be infused} \times \text{gtt/ml of administration set}}{\text{total time of infusion in minutes}}$$

e.g. You are instructed to administer 35 ml of IV fluid over 40 minutes using a microdrip administration set. *Your formula is: 35 ml × 60 gtt/ml = 2,100 gtt divided by 40 minutes = 52.5 gtt/minute (rounded to 50 gtt/minute) you need to administer.*

Intravenous Bolus Medications

<u>To complete this skill, do the following</u>:

1. Confirm medication order including drug name, dosage, and route.
2. Ask patient, "Do you have any known allergies?"
3. Select medication and make sure it is:
   - the correct drug and proper concentration.
   - clear.
   - not outdated.
4. Assemble prefilled syringe.
5. With needle pointed up, tap medication container until air bubbles rise to the top.
6. **Uncap needle and with it pointed up, dispel air so that only medication remains in the syringe**.
7. **Continue employing infection control precautions.** 😐
8. Cleanse medication injection site (Y-port or hub) of IV tubing.
9. Reconfirm name, concentration, and dosage of medication to be delivered.
10. Stop IV flow by pinching IV tubing above injection site.
11. **Administer correct dose of medication at proper push rate.**
12. **Flush IV tubing by briefly running it wide open or follow drug bolus with a 20 ml bolus of IV fluid**.
13. Adjust drip rate to a keep open rate (TKO, KVO).
14. **Dispose of syringe and needle (do not recap) in a proper biomedical waste container.** 😐
15. Observe patient for desired effect and adverse side effects. 😐 ⌦

Intravenous Piggyback Medications

To complete this skill, do the following:

1. Confirm medication order including drug name, dosage, and route. ☺
2. Ask patient, "Do you have any known allergies?"
3. Check selected IV fluid to make sure it is:
    - the proper solution.
    - clear.
    - not outdated.
    - not leaking.
4. **Select medication making sure it is correct drug, proper concentration,** clear, and not outdated.
5. Assemble prefilled syringe.
6. With needle pointed up, tap medication container until air bubbles rise to top.
7. Uncap needle and with it pointed up, dispel air so that only medication remains in syringe.
8. Continue employing infection control precautions.
9. Reconfirm that patient has no known allergies to medication.
10. Cleanse injection port of IV bag.
11. Invert bag and insert needle into rubber stopper of the injection port.
12. **Inject correct amount of medication** into IV solution and mix it by inverting IV bag several times.
13. Connect appropriate administration set to medication solution.
    - invert IV bag.

- using sterile techniques, insert spiked end of administration set into fluid port of IV bag.
- close off the flow control valve and turn IV bag right side up.
- squeeze drip chamber two or three times to fill it half way.
- **open the control valve to flush the tubing (to remove any air)**.

14. Attach an appropriate needle to the administration set (*typically* a 1 inch, 19 g. needle).
15. Continue employing infection control precautions.
16. Cleanse the medication port of the primary line closest to the patient.
17. Insert needle into medication port without contamination and tape it securely in place.
18. **Turn on flow of piggyback line and turn off primary IV**.
19. **Adjust flow rate of piggyback infusion to deliver correct dose**.
20. Observe patient for desired effect and adverse side effects. ☺ ⌦
21. Label medication/fluid bag with name and concentration of drug, time it was started and infusion rate (dosage per minute). ☺

Helpful Hints be sure to:

- ❑ **continually employ infection control procedures and dispose of your needles properly**.
- ❑ elevate the extremity after you administer IV bolus medications.
- ❑ **turn off the primary line when delivering an IV infusion**.
- ❑ observe the patient for the desired effects and adverse side effects.
- ❑ **begin IV bolus administration within 3 minutes and infusion medication within 5 minutes**.

■ math formulas for figuring IV flow rates, bolus, and IV infusions are shown on page 91.

Spinal Immobilization (seated patient)

To complete this skill, do the following:

1. Take infection control precautions. 😐
2. **Direct your partner or EMT assistant (from behind the patient) to place/maintain the patient's head in a neutral, in-line position**.
3. Assess your partner or EMT assistant's manual immobilization of the patient's head.
4. Assess motor, sensory, and distal circulation in all four of the patient's extremities. ⌦
5. Select an appropriately sized extrication collar and apply it without moving the patient.
6. Carefully move the patient forward and position the immobilization device behind him or her.
7. **Secure the immobilization device to the patient's torso so that it cannot move up or down, left or right**. When using a vest-type device, be sure that it is snug against the armpits. Typically, the chest straps are applied first, and then the groin straps. As you tighten the torso straps be careful not to jerk or move the patient unnecessarily.
8. Reevaluate the position and tightness of the torso straps (torso fixation), adjusting as necessary. ✓ to **ensure that chest expansion is not impaired by the tightness of the torso straps**.
9. **Evaluate and pad behind the patient's head as necessary**.
10. **Secure the patient's head to the device, being sure to maintain a neutral, in-line position.**
11. **Reassess motor, sensory, and distal circulation in all four extremities**.
12. Move the patient to a long backboard. 😐
    - move ambulance cot with a long backboard on it, perpendicular, next to car (vehicle) door opening.

- place end of long backboard next to or under the patient's buttock, so that one end is securely supported on the car seat and the other end on the ambulance cot.
- rotate patient (with the device in place) and elevate his or her legs.
- lower patient onto backboard and slide him or her up until properly positioned on the long backboard.
- lower patient's legs onto backboard (in some patients it may be necessary to loosen the groin straps).
- position long backboard onto ambulance cot.
- securely fasten device to the backboard.
- immobilize patient's legs to the long backboard.
- secure long backboard and patient to the cot.
- if the ambulance cot is not available, the long backboard can be held by others while the patient is lifted out of the seat and placed on the long backboard.

Helpful Hints be sure to:

- ❑ **immediately direct manual immobilization.**
- ❑ **avoid releasing manual immobilization before it is maintained with the immobilization device.**
- ❑ **secure the patient's head to the immobilization device only after the device has been secured to the torso.**
- ❑ **immobilize the head in a neutral, in-line position.**
- ❑ **avoid moving the patient excessively.**

Spinal Immobilization (lying patient)

To complete this skill, do the following:

1. Take (and direct your partners to) infection control procedures. ☹
2. **Direct your first partner or EMT assistant to move patient's head to a neutral, in-line position.**
3. **Then direct your EMT assistant to maintain manual immobilization of patient's head.**
4. Evaluate motor, sensory, and distal circulation in all four of the patient's extremities. ⌦
5. Apply a cervical collar and position a long backboard alongside patient.
6. Kneel next to patient's midthorax.
7. Direct your second partner or EMT assistant to kneel next to patient's knees.
8. Straighten patient's arms so that they are in a "palm-in" position next to the torso and direct your second partner or EMT assistant to bring the legs together into neutral alignment.
9. Grasp the far side of patient at his or her shoulder and wrist.
10. Direct your second partner or EMT assistant to grasp patient's hip with his or her left hand just distal to the wrist and tightly grasp both pant cuffs at the ankles with his or her right hand. (If patient is wearing shorts or a skirt, a cravat tied around both ankles can be used instead.)
11. Instruct your partners or EMT assistants when the patient is to be logrolled.
12. With patient's arms locked firmly at his or her sides, slowly roll the patient toward you until he or she is perpendicular to the ground. This must be done without compromising the integrity of the spine.
13. Position backboard close to patient, instruct your EMT assistants when patient is to be rolled back down.
14. Roll patient back onto long backboard. This must be done without compromising the integrity of the spine.

15. Keeping patient in neutral alignment, adjust patient's position so that he or she is centered on the board and proper space exists between the top of the board and patient's head.
16. Apply padding to voids between torso and long backboard as necessary.
17. **Immobilize patient's torso to long backboard so that it cannot move up or down or laterally.** Place one strap over nipple line and one strap over iliac crests.
18. **Evaluate and pad underneath patient's head as necessary.**
19. **Immobilize patient's head to the device** by placing pads or rolled blankets on each side of patient's head and fastening a strap tightly over pads and patient's lower forehead. Place a second strap over pads and rigid cervical collar and secure it to the long backboard.
20. Secure patient's legs to long backboard with one strap just above the knees and one strap midway between the ankles and knees.
21. Place patient's arms palm-in along his or her sides and secure them to long backboard.
22. **Reassess motor, sensory, and distal circulation.** ☺ ⌧

Helpful Hints be sure to:

- ❑ **immediately direct manual immobilization.**
- ❑ **avoid releasing manual immobilization before it is maintained with immobilization device.**
- ❑ **secure patient's head to immobilization device only after the device has been secured to the torso.**
- ❑ **avoid moving patient excessively.**

Bleeding – Wounds – Shock

To complete this skill, do the following:

1. **Employ infection control precautions.** 😐
2. Apply direct pressure to the wound with a gloved hand.
3. Elevate the wound (if it is on an extremity).
4. Apply a pressure dressing to the wound.
5. Bandage the wound.
6. Apply additional dressings if the wound continues to bleed.
7. Locate and apply pressure to the appropriate arterial pressure point if the wound continues to bleed.
8. If the injury mechanism or signs indicate the victim is in compensatory shock:
    - **apply a high concentration of oxygen.**
    - properly position the patient (supine with his or her legs elevated).
    - prevent heat loss (cover the patient as appropriate).
9. If the injury mechanism or signs indicate the victim is in profound shock:
    - remove clothing or check for sharp objects. 😐 ⌧
    - quickly perform a secondary assessment of the areas of the body that will be covered by the PASG. ⌧
    - **position the PASG with the top of the abdominal section at or below the lowest ribs.**
    - secure the PASG around the patient.
    - attach the hoses, open the stopcocks, and inflate the PASG until: 😐 ⌧
        - the patient's systolic blood pressure returns to above 100 mm Hg

   - or the Velcro begins to crackle or pop-off valves release air.
- **✓ the patient's blood pressure and vital signs.**
- **close off the stopcocks to maintain the air pressure in the garment.**

10. Reassess the patient's vital signs. ☺ ⌦

Helpful Hints be sure to:

- ❑ **take or verbalize infection control precautions.**
- ❑ **apply a tourniquet only after applying all other methods of bleeding control if bleeding is still occurring.**
- ❑ **position the garment below the level of the lowest rib.**
- ❑ prevent the garment from causing respiratory embarrassment.
- ❑ secure the garment so that it fits snugly around the patient's extremities and abdomen.
- ❑ face all valves and hoses outward when applied.
- ❑ maintain appropriate spinal column immobilization.
- ❑ **administer a high concentration of oxygen.**
- ❑ **reassess vital signs after inflation of the PASG.**
- ❑ **close off the stopcocks to maintain the air pressure in the garment.**
- ❑ **inflate the legs before or at the same time as the abdomen.**

Long Bone Fracture Immobilization (radius, ulna)

To complete this skill, do the following:

1. Take infection control precautions. ☺
2. Direct your partner or EMT assistant to apply manual stabilization.
3. Assess motor, sensory, and distal circulation in the injured extremity. ⌦
4. **Immobilize patient's hand in position of function**. To accomplish this the wrist should be dorsiflexed about 20-30° and all fingers flexed slightly. This is the position in which one most comfortably holds a baseball. Then place a soft roller bandage into the palm of the patient's hand.
5. Measure the splint and immobilize joint below the fracture by applying the splint to the palmar side of the hand and wrist. Secure it with a soft roller bandage throughout the length of the splint, **making sure above and below the fracture are immobilized**.
6. **Secure the entire injured extremity by applying a sling and swath**. A pillow may be placed between the arm and chest for patient comfort.
7. **Reassess motor, sensory, and distal circulation in the injured extremity**. ⌦

Helpful Hints be sure to:

- ❑ **handle the injured extremity carefully—do not allow gross movement**.
- ❑ **immobilize adjacent joints**.
- ❑ **✓ motor, sensory, and distal circulation of the injured extremity before and after splinting**.
- ❑ avoid applying the splint too tightly or too loosely.

Long Bone Fracture Immobilization (tibia, fibula)

To complete this skill, do the following:

1. Take infection control precautions, cut the trouser leg to expose the injury site, and remove the shoe and sock.* ☺ ⌦
2. Direct your partner or EMT assistant to apply manual stabilization.
3. Assess motor, sensory, and distal circulation in the injured extremity. ☺ ⌦
4. Measure the splint(s).
5. Place one padded board splint medially and one laterally.
6. Pad the voids.
7. **Immobilize the joint above and below the fracture**.
8. **Immobilize the foot in the position of function**.
9. Secure the entire injured extremity by placing the patient onto a long backboard. ☺
10. **Reassess motor, sensory, and distal circulation in the injured extremity**. ⌦

Helpful Hints be sure to:

- ❑ **handle the injured extremity carefully—do not allow gross movement**.
- ❑ **immobilize adjacent joints**.
- ❑ **✓ motor, sensory, and distal circulation before and after splinting**.
- ❑ avoid applying the splint too tightly or too loosely.

Traction Splinting (Hare traction splint)

To complete this skill, do the following:

1. Take infection control precautions, cut the trouser leg to expose the injury site, and remove the shoe and sock. * ☺ ⌦
2. Direct your partner or EMT assistant to apply manual stabilization to the injured leg so that no motion occurs at the fracture site.
3. Direct your partner or EMT assistant to apply manual traction.
4. Assess motor, sensory, and distal circulation in the injured extremity. ⌦
5. Apply the ankle hitch.*
6. Measure the splint against the good leg (typically the pad is at the ischial tuberosity and the end of the splint extends approximately 8-12 inches beyond the foot).
7. Position the splint at the injured leg.
8. Open and adjust the four Velcro support straps (mid-thigh, above the knee, below the knee, and above the ankle).*
9. While your partner or EMT assistant lifts the injured leg, apply the splint by sliding it under the patient's injured limb so that the ischial pad is seated well against the ischial tuberosity.
10. **Gently apply the proximal ischial strap**.
11. With your partner or EMT assistant maintaining gentle manual traction on the patient's injured extremity, connect the "S" hook of the ratchet mechanism (of the splint) to the loops of the ankle hitch.

12. Apply mechanical traction; continue until the patient's pain is relieved **without releasing manual traction**. ☹
13. Secure the splint support straps around the leg and release manual traction if mechanical traction is adequate.
14. Re-evaluate proximal/distal securing devices. ⌦
15. **Reassess motor, sensory, and distal circulation**. ⌦
16. Secure the patient to a long backboard: ☹
    - logroll the patient onto the board.
    - secure the patient's torso to a long backboard to immobilize the hip.
    - secure the splint to the long backboard to prevent movement of the splint.

Helpful Hints be sure to:

- ❑ **keep traction at all times once it has been applied**.
- ❑ **reassess motor, sensory, and distal circulation after splinting**.
- ❑ **avoid rotating or extending the foot**.
- ❑ **apply the ischial strap before applying mechanical traction**.
- ❑ avoid applying supporting straps over the knee or fracture site.
- ❑ avoid applying the supporting straps too tightly.
- ❑ avoid applying too much mechanical traction.

Section 3

ECG characteristics
Sample case history with treatment

ECG Dysrhythmia Interpretation Skills

Described below is a brief review of how to interpret ECG dysrhythmias.

To analyze ECG dysrhythmias, look at the following:

- ***Rhythm*** *(is it regular or irregular?)*
- ***Rate*** *(is it normal, fast, slow?)*
- ***P waves*** *(is there an upright, uniform P wave preceding each QRS complex?)*
- ***P-R intervals*** *(are P-R intervals identifiable? within normal limits [0.12-0.20 seconds]? constant in duration?)*
- ***QRS complexes*** *(are the QRS complexes within normal limits [≤0.10 seconds]? do they appear normal?)*

  (Some texts use ≤0.10 seconds, some use <0.12 seconds. Both are acceptable.)

The information gathered, using the format listed above, is matched against characteristics common to the various cardiac dysrhythmias. This provides you with the information needed to interpret ECG dysrhythmias.

In this section, the ECGs are organized according to their primary characteristics and not the more traditional format of listing them by their origin (e.g., atrial, junctional, ventricular dysrhythmias). We use this format to make it easier to locate key information about the various dysrhythmias. At the bottom of each ECG page, highlighted in reverse type (white lettering on black background), are key characteristics.

This makes it even easier to spot information in a hurry. We have also provided longer ECG strips to give you clearer examples of the various dysrhythmias. While sitting in the ECG station you now have instant access to the ECG characteristics common to the various dysrhythmias.

In this section of the guide, dysrhythmias are organized according to the format described above:

Rate *(slow rates including: sinus bradycardia, junctional escape, 2nd-degree AV heart block, 3rd-degree AV heart block, idioventricular rhythm, asystole and fast rates including: sinus tachycardia, PSVT, ventricular tachycardia).*
Rhythm *(irregular rhythms including: PACs, PJCs, PVCs, ventricular fibrillation).*
Noncharacteristic P waves, P-R intervals or QRS complexes *(atrial flutter, atrial fibrillation).*

While not every dysrhythmia is shown in this booklet, every effort has been made to include the major concepts of dysrhythmia interpretation.

The design of this book places cardiac treatments in a section close to the ECG dysrhythmias section. This allows you to easily look at the ECGs and their recommended treatments. Treatments for PEA, acute myocardial infarction, CHF, acute pulmonary edema, and shock are listed at the end of the treatment section.

Also included at the end of this section is a sample case history with the suggested treatment. This sample case gives you a sense of what to expect in the static ECG dysrhythmia testing station of the National Registry and state certification exams.

Normal Sinus Rhythm

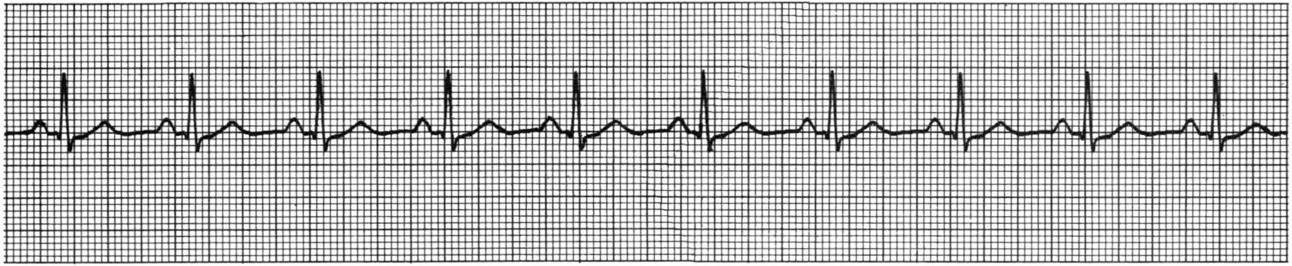

Look for these characteristics

Rhythm	Regular (R-R intervals and P-P intervals are constant).
Rate	60 to 100 per minute (atrial and ventricular rates are equal).
P Waves	Upright and uniform, precede each QRS complex.
P-R Intervals	Within normal limits (0.12-0.20 seconds in duration) and constant.
QRS Complexes	Within normal limits (≤0.10 seconds in duration).

The following pages list the characteristics of

SLOW HEART RATES

Sinus Bradycardia

(treatment for this dysrhythmia listed on page 63)

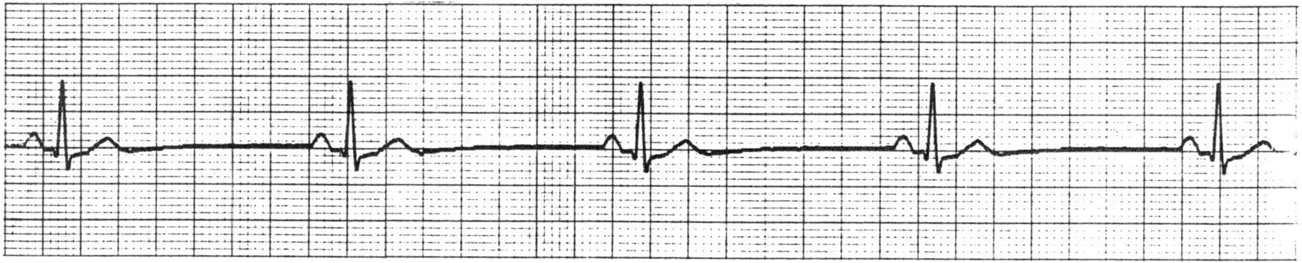

Look for these characteristics

Rhythm	Regular (R-R intervals and P-P intervals are constant).
Rate	<60 beats per minute.
P Waves	Upright and uniform, precede each QRS complex.
P-R Intervals	Within normal limits (0.12-0.20 seconds) and constant.
QRS Complexes	Within normal limits (≤0.10 seconds).

SLOW RATE, narrow QRS complexes, uniform P waves

Junctional Escape Rhythm

(treatment for this dysrhythmia listed on page 63)

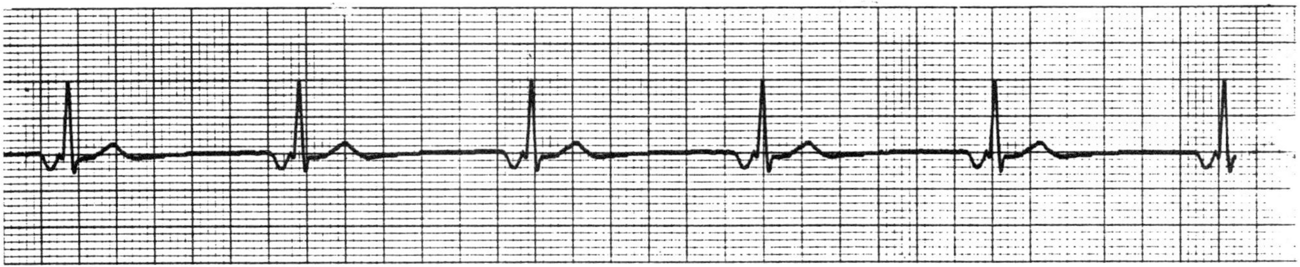

<u>Look for these characteristics</u>

Rhythm	Regular.
Rate	Between 40 to 60 beats per minute.
P Waves	May precede, be lost in (absent), or follow the QRS complex. When present, the P wave will be inverted.
P-R Intervals	If present, it will be <0.12 seconds and constant.
QRS Complexes	Within normal limits (≤0.10 seconds).

SLOW RATE, narrow QRS complexes, inverted or absent P waves

2nd-Degree AV Heart Block, Wenckebach

(treatment listed on page 63)

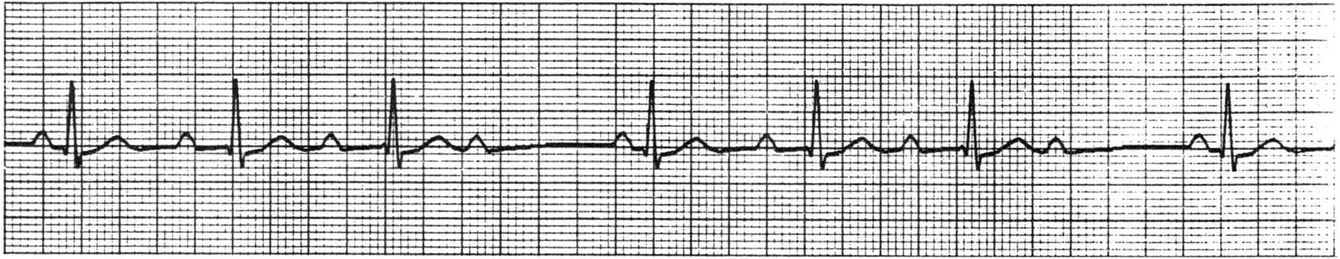

<u>Look for these characteristics</u>

Rhythm	Irregular, appears as a pattern (cycle seems to occur over and over again).
Rate	Ventricular rate is slightly slower than normal.
P Waves	Upright and uniform, there are more P waves than QRS complexes as some of the QRS complexes are blocked.
P-R Intervals	Get progressively longer until a QRS complex is "dropped." After the blocked beat, the cycle starts all over again.
QRS Complexes	Within normal limits (≤0.10 seconds).

SLOW RATE, irregular rhythm, more P waves than QRS complexes, varying P-R intervals

2nd-Degree AV Heart Block, Mobitz II

(treatment for this dysrhythmia listed on page 63)

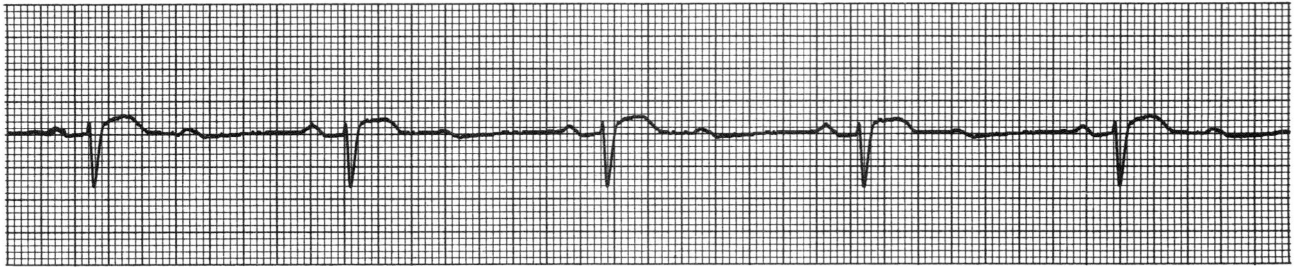

Look for these characteristics

Rhythm Typically regular. Is irregular if the conduction ratio (number of P waves to each QRS complex) varies.

Rate The ventricular rate is slower than normal (<60 beats per minute) while the atrial rate is within normal range.

P Waves Upright and uniform. There are more P waves than QRS complexes.

P-R Intervals Constant, can be normal or longer than normal (>0.20 seconds).

QRS Complexes Within normal limits (≤0.10 seconds).

SLOW RATE, more P waves than QRS complexes, constant PR intervals

3rd-Degree AV Heart Block (complete)

(treatment for this dysrhythmia listed on page 63)

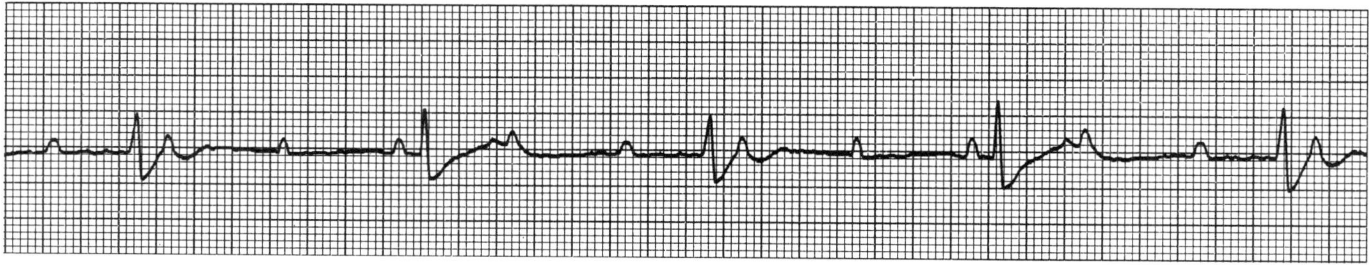

Look for these characteristics

Rhythm	Regular.
Rate	The ventricular rate is slower than normal (<60 beats per minute) while the atrial rate is within normal range.
P Waves	There are more P waves than QRS complexes.
P-R Intervals	There is no relationship between the P waves and QRS complexes, "the P waves seem to march right through the QRS complexes."
QRS Complexes	May be normal or wide, is dependent upon how low in the conduction pathway the escape beats are.

SLOW RATE, P waves march through the QRS complexes

Idioventricular Rhythm (Ventricular Escape)

(treatment listed on page 63 used **when pulse is present**)
(treatment listed on page 62 used **when pulse is absent**)

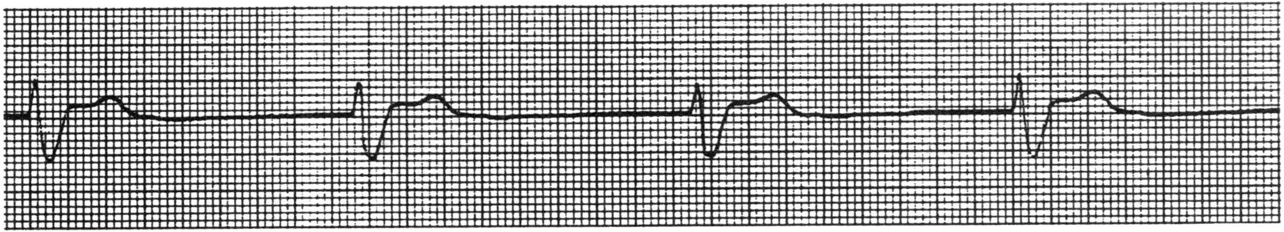

Look for these characteristics

Rhythm	Regular (becomes irregular as the heart dies).
Rate	<40 beats per minute.
P Waves	Absent.
P-R Intervals	Absent.
QRS Complexes	Wide (>0.10 seconds) and bizarre, the T wave typically takes the opposite direction of the R wave.

SLOW RATE, wide QRS complexes, no P waves

Asystole

(treatment for this dysrhythmia listed on page 62)

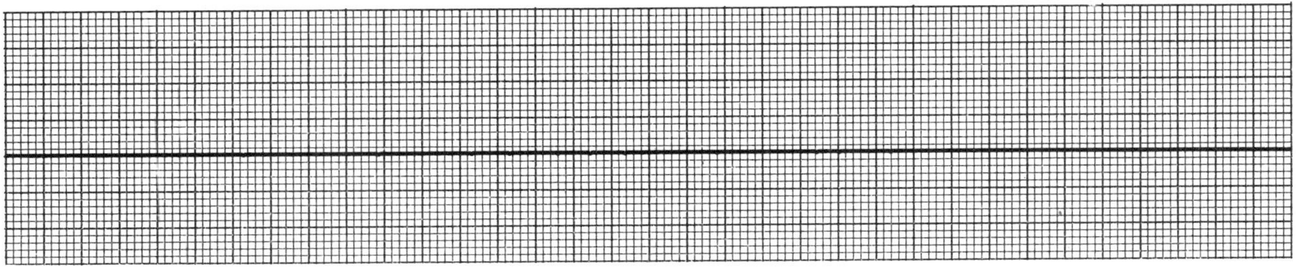

Look for these characteristics

Rhythm	Absent.
Rate	Absent.
P Waves	There is no electrical activity, only a flat line.
P-R Intervals	There is no electrical activity, only a flat line.
QRS Complexes	There is no electrical activity, only a flat line.

FLATLINE (absence of a rhythm)

The following pages list the characteristics of

FAST HEART RATES

Sinus Tachycardia

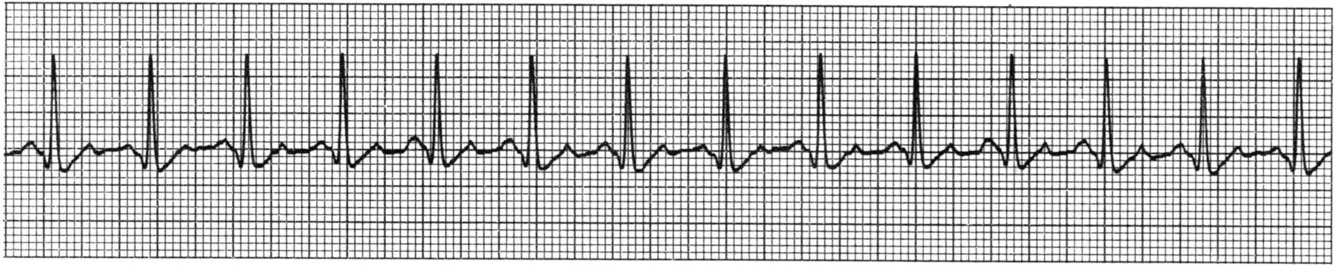

Look for these characteristics

Rhythm	Regular (R-R intervals and P-P intervals are constant).
Rate	Between 100 and 160 beats per minute.
P Waves	Upright and uniform, precede each QRS complex.
P-R Intervals	Within normal limits (0.12-0.20 seconds) and constant.
QRS Complexes	Within normal limits (≤0.10 seconds).

FAST RATE, narrow QRS complexes, uniform P waves

Paroxysmal Supraventricular Tachycardia (PSVT)

(treatment for this dysrhythmia listed on pages 64 and 65)

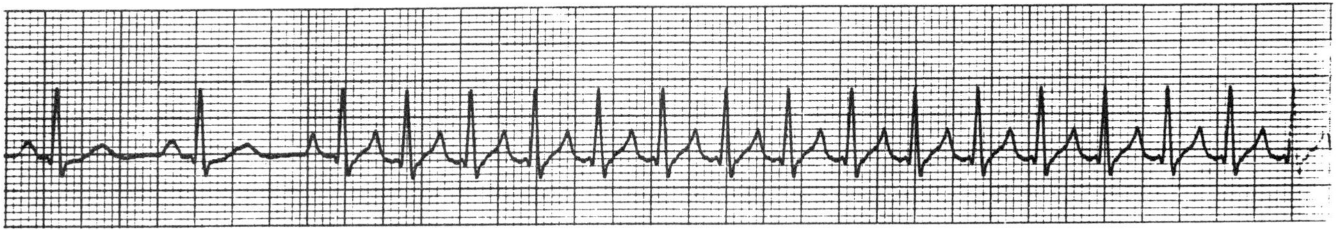

Look for these characteristics

Rhythm	Regular.
Rate	Usually >160 beats per minute.
P Waves	There is one P wave preceding each QRS complex. The P wave is typically buried in the T wave of the preceding beat. If present, the P waves may be flattened or notched.
P-R Intervals	Because the P waves tend to be buried, the intervals are typically indeterminable. If present, they will be within normal limits.
QRS Complexes	Typically within normal limits (≤0.10 seconds).

Ventricular Tachycardia

(treatment for this dysrhythmia listed on pages 64 and 65)

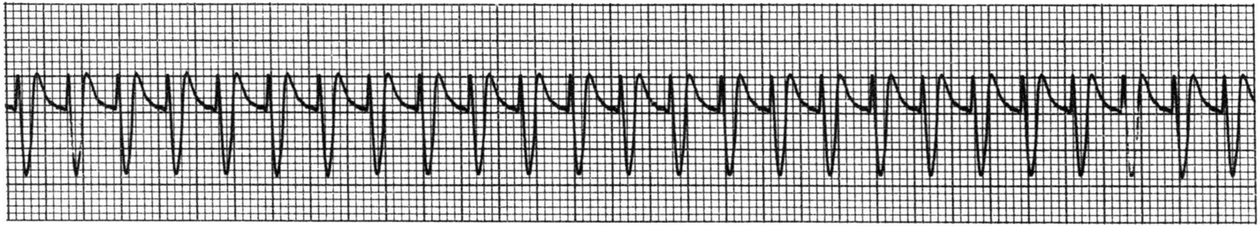

Look for these characteristics

Rhythm Typically regular.

Rate Ventricular rate is between 150-250 beats per minute. If the rate is <150 it is referred to as slow VT. If the rate is >250 it is referred to as ventricular flutter.

P Waves Typically absent (if seen, they are dissociated).

P-R Intervals Absent.

QRS Complexes Wide (>0.10 seconds) and bizarre. T waves of the ventricular beats take an opposite direction to the R waves. Beats are usually followed by a compensatory pulse.

FAST RATE, wide QRS complexes, P waves absent

The following pages list the characteristics of

Premature Atrial Complexes (PACs)

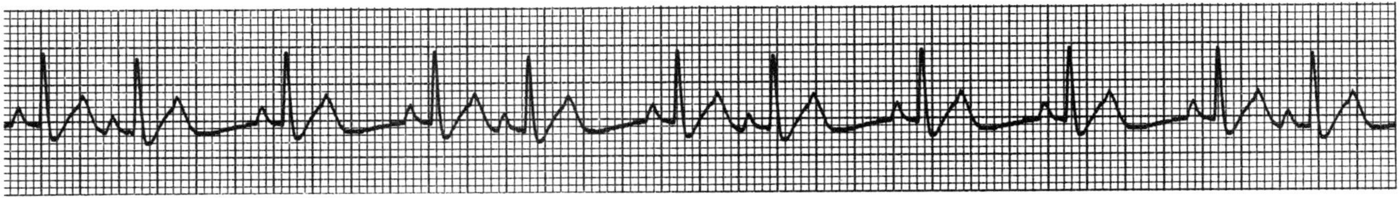

Look for these characteristics

Rhythm	Irregular (underlying rhythm is disrupted by presence of early beats).
Rate	Is dependent on the rate of the underlying rhythm.
P Waves	Present with the underlying rhythm and premature beats.
P-R Intervals	Present with the underlying rhythm and premature beats, is within normal limits.
QRS Complexes	Premature beats are narrow (≤0.10 seconds) and look the same as QRS complexes of the underlying rhythm. T waves of the premature beats are of the same direction as the R waves. PACs are not usually followed by a compensatory pause.

IRREGULAR RHYTHM, early beats with narrow QRS complexes, P waves present

Premature Junctional Complexes (PJCs)

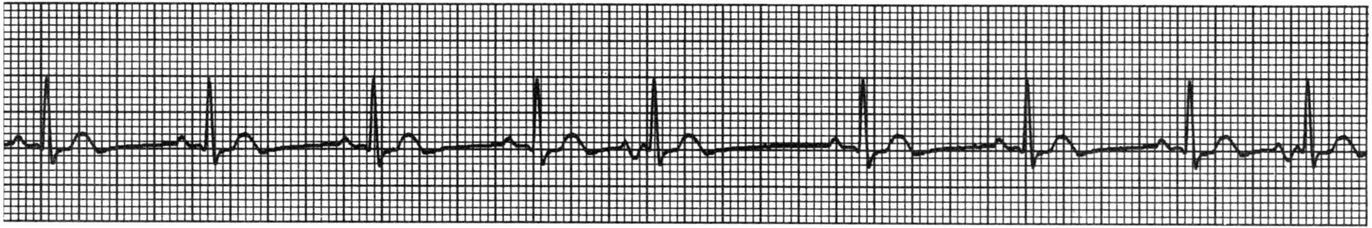

Look for these characteristics

Rhythm	Irregular (underlying rhythm is disrupted by presence of early beats).
Rate	Is dependent on the rate of the underlying rhythm.
P Waves	Typically present with the underlying rhythm but not the premature beats. If present, the P waves are usually inverted.
P-R Intervals	Typically present with the underlying rhythm. If present with the premature beats, will be <0.12 seconds.
QRS Complexes	Premature beats are narrow (≤0.10 seconds) and look the same as QRS complexes of the underlying rhythm. T waves of the premature beats are of the same direction as the R waves. PJCs are not usually followed by a compensatory pulse.

IRREGULAR RHYTHM, early beats with narrow QRS complexes, inverted or absent P waves

Premature Ventricular Complexes (PVCs) (treatment for this dysrhythmia listed on page 56)

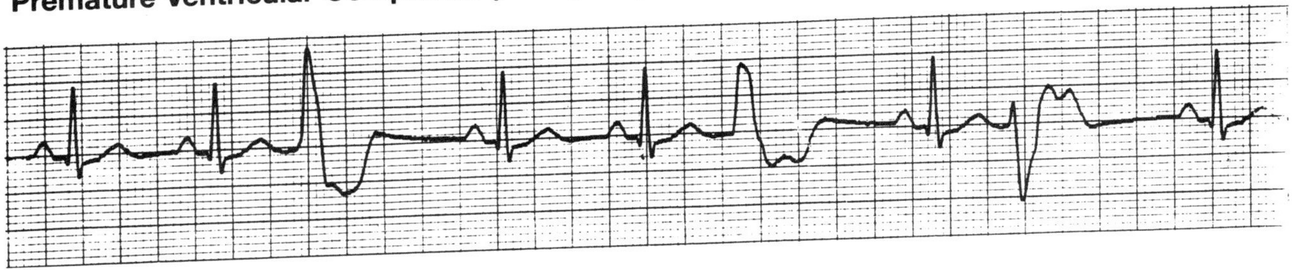

Look for these characteristics

Rhythm Irregular (underlying rhythm is disrupted by presence of the early beats).

Rate Is dependent on the rate of the underlying rhythm.

P Waves Typically present with the underlying rhythm but not the premature beats.

P-R Intervals Typically present with the underlying rhythm but not the premature beats.

QRS Complexes Premature beats are wide (>0.10 seconds) and bizarre, and differ from QRS complexes of the underlying rhythm. T waves of the premature beats take an opposite direction to the R waves. PVCs usually followed by a complete compensatory pause.

IRREGULAR RHYTHM, early beats with wide, bizarre QRS complexes, P waves absent

Ventricular Fibrillation

(treatment for this dysrhythmia listed on pages 60 and 61)

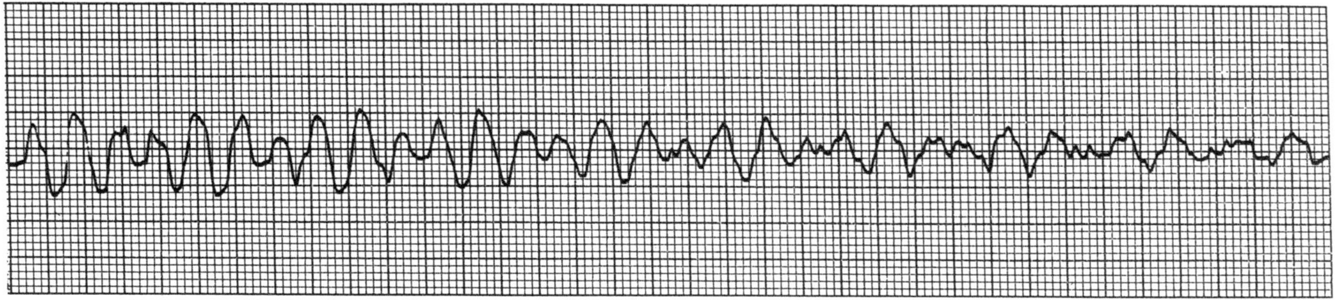

Look for these characteristics

Rhythm Totally chaotic.
Rate Cannot be determined as there are no discernible waves to measure.
P Waves There are no discernible P waves.
P-R Intervals There are no intervals.
QRS Complexes There are no discernible QRS complexes.

CHAOTIC RHYTHM with no uniform wave forms

RHYTHMS WITHOUT P WAVES

The following pages list the characteristics of

Atrial Flutter

(treatment for this dysrhythmia listed on pages 64 and 65)

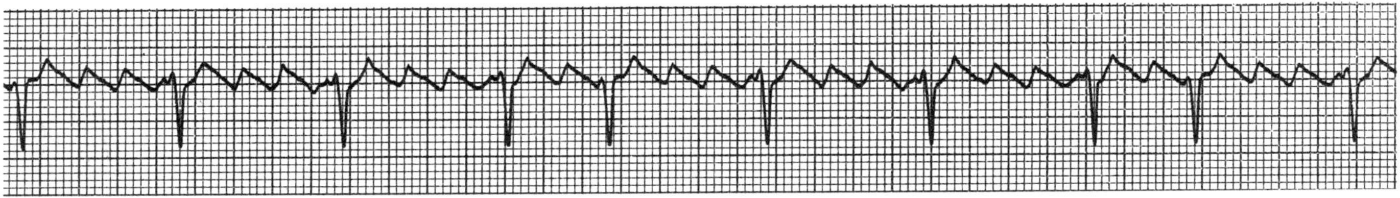

<u>Look for these characteristics</u>

Rhythm	Atrial rhythm is regular; depending on conduction ratio, ventricular rhythm may be regular or irregular.
Rate	Depends on ventricular response, may be normal, slow or fast.
P Waves	There are no discernible P waves. The atrial activity is represented by "flutter waves" which produce a characteristic "sawtooth appearance."
P-R Intervals	Absent.
QRS Complexes	Within normal limits (≤0.10 seconds).

P WAVES REPLACED BY FLUTTER WAVES

Atrial Fibrillation

(treatment for this dysrhythmia listed on pages 64 and 65)

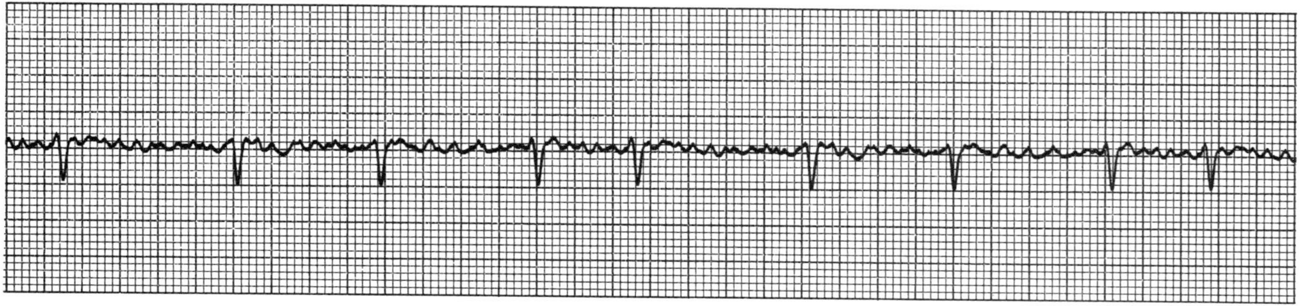

Look for these characteristics

Rhythm	Totally (grossly) irregular. Also referred to as irregularly irregular.
Rate	Depends on ventricular response, may be normal, slow, or fast.
P Waves	There are no discernible P waves, the baseline is chaotic as the atrial activity is represented by "fibrillatory waves."
P-R Intervals	Absent.
QRS Complexes	Within normal limits (≤0.10 seconds).

FIBRILLATORY ATRIAL WAVE FORMS, totally irregular rhythm

Pulseless Electrical Activity (PEA)

(treatment for this dysrhythmia listed on page 62)

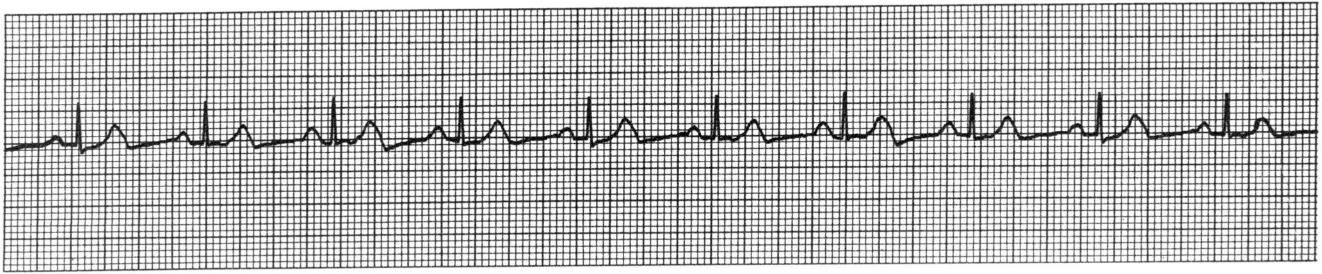

Look for these characteristics

Rhythm	May be regular or irregular.
Rate	May be fast, normal or slow.
P Waves	May be present or absent, depends on origin of rhythm.
P-R Intervals	May be present or absent, depends on origin of rhythm.
QRS Complexes	May be normal width or wide and bizarre (>0.10 seconds), depends on rhythm origin.
Additional Information	The primary characteristic associated with this condition is the presence of an electrical rhythm without a corresponding pulse. The electrical activity may appear as sinus rhythm, sinus tachycardia, idioventricular rhythm, or other rhythms. PEA includes electro-mechanical dissociation (EMD), pseudo-EMD, idioventricular rhythms, ventricular escape rhythms, bradyasystolic rhythms, or post defibrillation idioventricular rhythms.

REGULAR RHYTHM, no pulse

Sample Case History

Your patient is a 48-year-old female who experienced syncope while bowling. She is confused, has a blood pressure of 142/90 and cold, diaphoretic skin. Estimated weight is 100 kg. You attach the patient to the ECG monitor and see the dysrhythmia shown on page 51.

Sample Treatment for Premature Ventricular Complexes

- OXYGEN
- RULE OUT treatable cause; consider:
  - *electrolyte imbalance (hypokalemia, hypomagnesemia)*
  - *digitalis level*
  - *bradycardia*
  - *drugs*
- LIDOCAINE, 1-1.5 mg/kg, IV push, followed by LIDOCAINE, 2-4 mg/min, IV infusion

<u>If PVCs persist</u>:

Repeat LIDOCAINE, 0.5-0.75 mg/kg every 2-5 min until no ectopy, or up to 3 mg/kg

<u>Consider</u>:

- PROCAINAMIDE
- OVERDRIVE PACING

Section 4

ACLS treatment algorithms

Special Information

- dosage-related treatments (medications, defibrillation) are **bolded** for easy visualization.
- questions you should ask are identified by **shaded triangles**.
- conditions that you determine the patient to be in are identified by **shaded boxes**.
- references to other critical information are identified by the "📖" **symbol** followed by a page number (that identifies the first page where the information can be found).

Universal Algorithm

Starting point for all patient assessment.

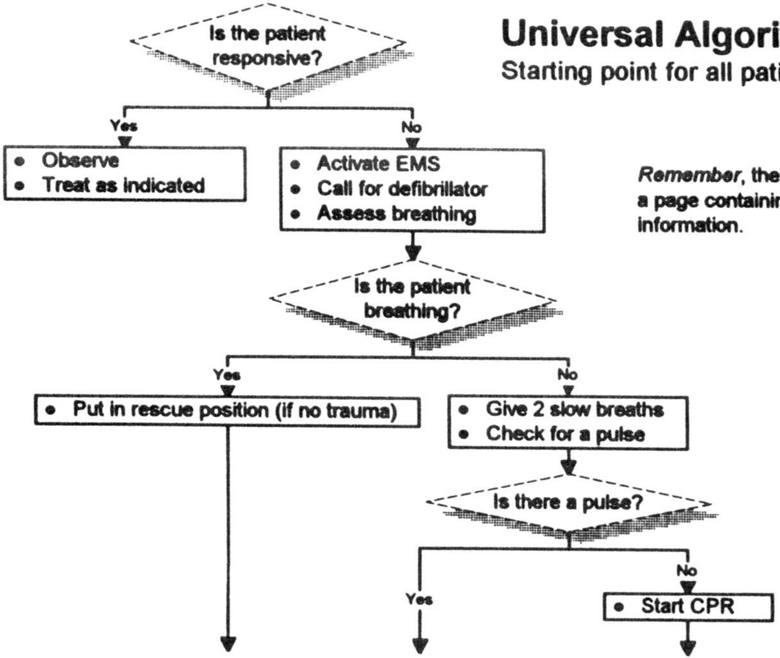

Remember, the 🕮 symbol refers you to a page containing important reference information.

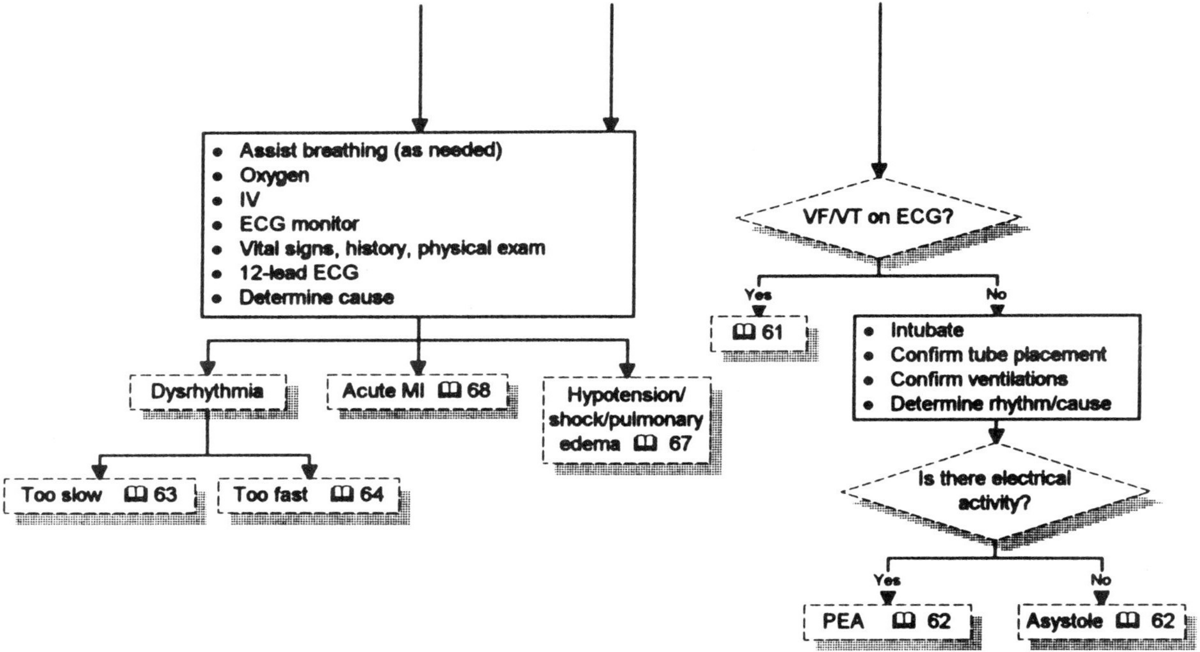

Assist breathing (as needed)
Oxygen
IV
ECG monitor
Vital signs, history, physical exam
12-lead ECG
Determine cause
Dysrhythmia
Acute MI 68
Hypotension/ shock/pulmonary edema 67
Too slow 63
Too fast 64
VF/VT on ECG?
Yes
No
61
Intubate
Confirm tube placement
Confirm ventilations
Determine rhythm/cause
Is there electrical activity?
Yes
No
PEA 62
Asystole 62

Ventricular Fibrillation/ Tachycardia

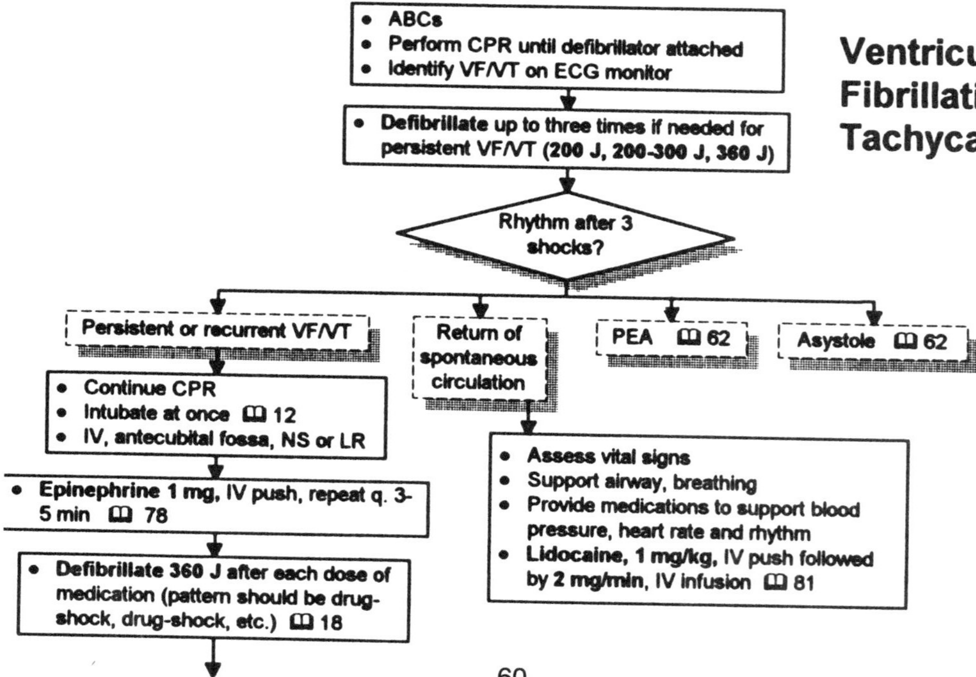

Continue by administering medications of probable benefit.

↓

- **Lidocaine, 1.5 mg/kg,** IV push (repeat in 3-5 min to a total dose of 3 mg/kg) 📖 81

↓

- **Defibrillate 360 J** 📖 18

↓

- **Bretylium, 5 mg/kg,** IV push (repeat in 5 min at 10 mg/kg to a total of 30-35 mg/kg) 📖 72

↓

- **Defibrillate 360 J** 📖 18

↓

<u>Consider use of</u>:

- **Magnesium Sulfate, 1-2 grams,** IV push 📖 82
- **Procainamide, 30 mg/min,** IV push (total of 17 mg/kg) 📖 88
- **Sodium Bicarbonate, 1 mEq/kg,** IV push 📖 89

↓

- **Defibrillate 360 J** 📖 18

↓

- Continue CPR

Asystole

Pulseless Electrical Activity (PEA)

- Continue CPR
- Intubate at once
- IV, antecubital fossa, NS or LR

Asystole

- Confirm asystole in more than one lead

↓

Consider possible causes

- Hypoxia
- Hyperkalemia 📖 73
- Hypokalemia
- Preexisting acidosis 📖 89
- Drug overdose
- Hypothermia

↓

- Consider immediate transcutaneous pacing (TCP)

↓

- Epinephrine, 1 mg, IV push, repeat q. 3-5 min 📖 78

↓

- Atropine, 1 mg, IV push, repeat q. 3-5 min up to a total of 0.04 mg/kg 📖 71

↓

- Consider termination of efforts

Pulseless Electrical Activity (PEA)

- Assess blood flow using Doppler ultrasound

↓

Consider possible causes

- Hypovolemia (volume infusion)
- Hypoxia (oxygen, ventilation)
- Cardiac tamponade (pericardiocentesis)
- Tension pneumothorax (needle decompression)
- Massive pulmonary embolism (surgery, thrombolytics)
- Hyperkalemia 📖 73
- Acidosis 📖 89
- Drug overdose such as tricyclics, digitalis, β-blockers, calcium channel blockers
- Hypothermia
- Massive AMI 📖 68

↓

- Epinephrine, 1 mg, IV push, repeat q. 3-5 min 📖 78

↓

- If absolute (<60 beats/min) or relative bradycardia give atropine, 1 mg, IV push, repeat q. 3-5 min up to a total of 0.04 mg/kg 📖 71

Bradycardia

<u>Serious symptoms and signs include</u>: chest pain, dyspnea, decreased level of consciousness, hypotension, shock, pulmonary congestion, CHF, acute MI.

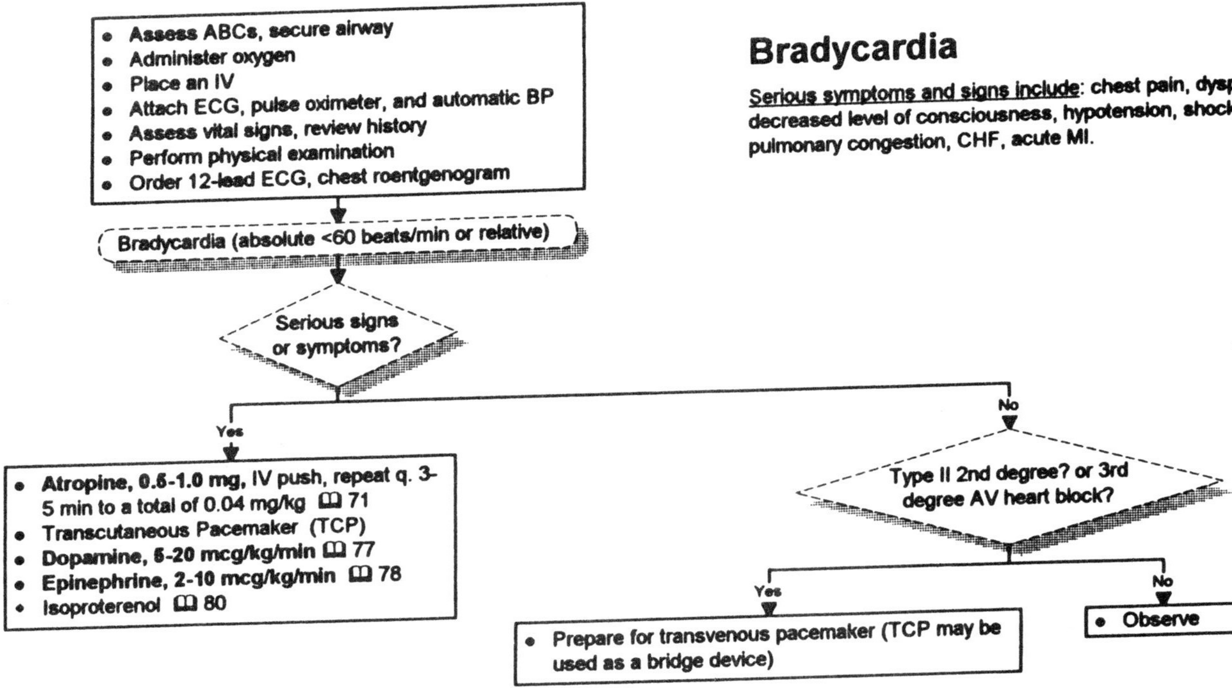

Tachycardia

Serious signs and symptoms include: chest pain, dyspnea, decreased level of consciousness, hypotension, shock, pulmonary congestion, CHF, acute MI.

- Assess ABCs, secure airway, administer oxygen
- Prepare intubation equipment
- Place an IV
- Attach ECG, pulse oximeter, and automatic BP
- Assess vital signs, review history
- Perform physical examination
- Order 12-lead ECG, chest roentgenogram

↓

Serious signs or symptoms?

Yes →

If VT, PSVT, atrial fibrillation/flutter and ventricular rate is > 150 beats per minute:

- **Deliver immediate synchronized cardioversion at 100 J, 200 J, 300 J, 360 J** (premedicate whenever possible)
- May give brief trial of medications in certain rhythms

No (or borderline) ↓

Atrial fibrillation/flutter

Consider use of:
- **Diltiazem** 📖 75
- **β-Blockers**
- **Verapamil**
- **Digoxin**
- **Procainamide**
- **Quinidine**
- **Anticoagulants**

Paroxysmal supraventricular tachycardia (PSVT)

- Vagal maneuvers

↓

- **Adenosine, 6 mg, rapid IV push**

↓

If unresolved in 1-2 min:
- **Adenosine, 12 mg**, rapid IV push. May repeat once in 1-2 min 📖 70

↓

Wide-complex tachycardia (uncertain type)

- **Lidocaine, 1-1.5 mg/kg**, IV push 📖 81

↓

If unresolved:
- **Lidocaine, 0.5-0.75 mg/kg**, IV push. Repeat q. 5-10 min to a total of 3 mg/kg

↓

Ventricular tachycardia (VT)

- **Lidocaine, 1-1.5 mg/kg**, IV push 📖 81

↓

If unresolved:
- **Lidocaine, 0.5-0.75 mg/kg**, IV push. Repeat q. 5-10 min to a total of 3 mg/ kg

↓

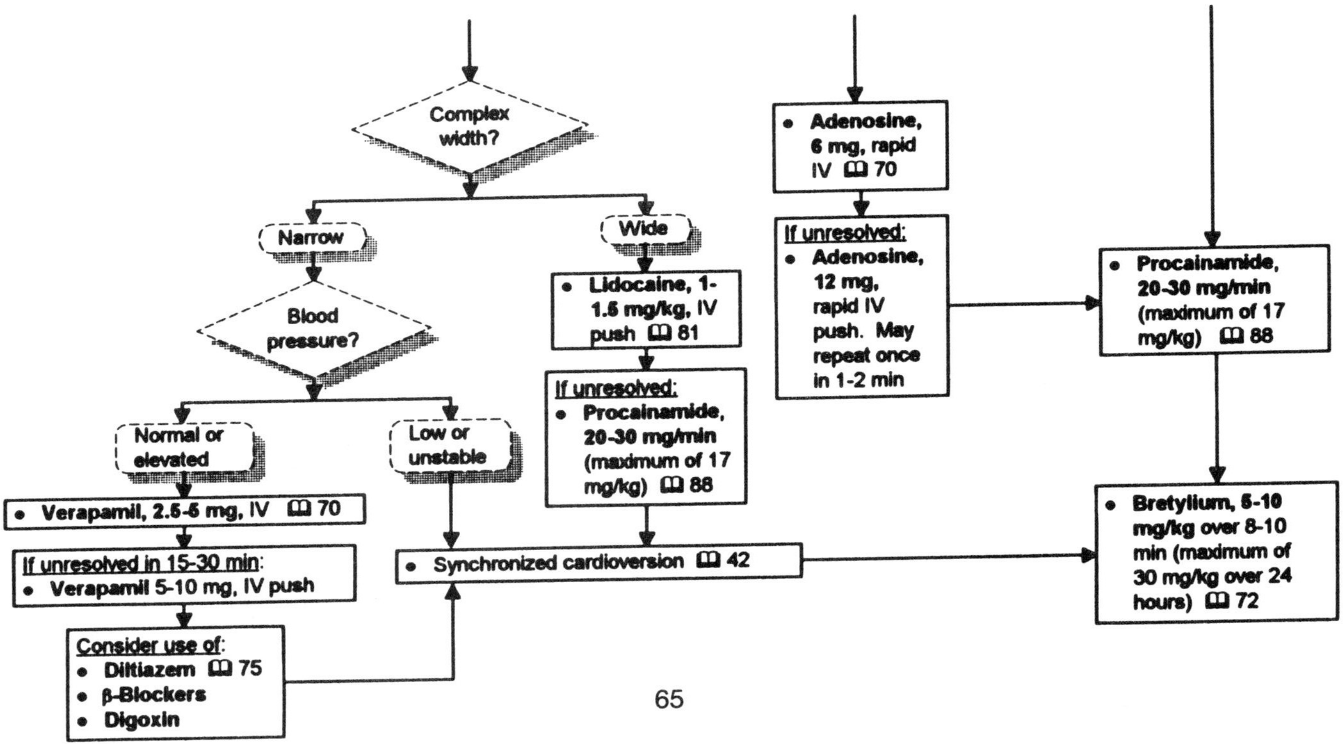
Complex width?
Narrow
Wide
Blood pressure?
Normal or elevated
Low or unstable
• Verapamil, 2.5-5 mg, IV 70
If unresolved in 15-30 min:
• Verapamil 5-10 mg, IV push
Consider use of:
• Diltiazem 75
• β-Blockers
• Digoxin
• Lidocaine, 1-1.5 mg/kg, IV push 81
If unresolved:
• Procainamide, 20-30 mg/min (maxmum of 17 mg/kg) 88
• Synchronized cardioversion 42
• Adenosine, 6 mg, rapid IV 70
If unresolved:
• Adenosine, 12 mg, rapid IV push. May repeat once in 1-2 min
• Procainamide, 20-30 mg/min (maximum of 17 mg/kg) 88
• Bretylium, 5-10 mg/kg over 8-10 min (maximum of 30 mg/kg over 24 hours) 72

Hypotension, Shock and Acute Pulmonary Edema

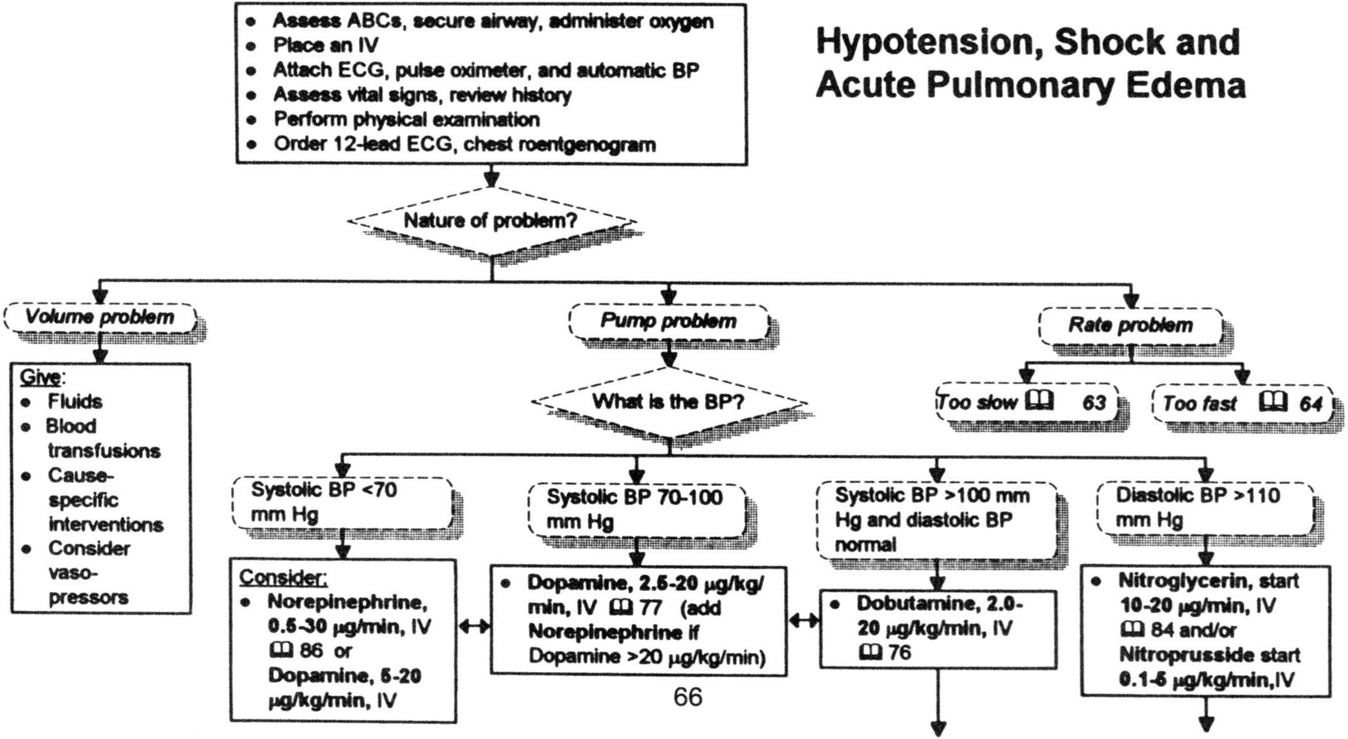

Consider additional treatments, especially if acute pulmonary edema is present

<u>First-line actions</u>

- **Furosemide, 0.5-1.0 mg/kg, IV** 📖 79
- **Morphine, 1-3 mg, IV** 📖 83
- **Nitroglycerin**, SL
- **Oxygen/intubate** PRN

<u>Second-line actions</u>

- **Nitroglycerin** IV (if BP >100 mm Hg)
- **Nitroprusside** IV (if BP >100 mmHg) 📖 85
- **Dopamine** (if BP <100 mm Hg)
- **Dobutamine** (if BP >100 mm Hg)
- Positive end-expiratory pressure (PEEP)
- Continuous positive airway pressure (CPAP)

<u>Third-line actions</u>

- **Amrinone, 0.75 mg/kg then 5-15 μg/kg per min, IV** (if other drugs fail)
- **Aminophylline, 5.0 mg/kg** (if wheezing)
- **Thrombolytic therapy** (if not in shock)
- **Digoxin** (if atrial fibrillation, supraventricular tachycardia)
- Angioplasty (if drugs fail)
- Intra-aortic balloon pump (bridge to surgery)
- Surgical interventions (valves, coronary artery bypass grafts, heart transplant, etc.)

Acute Myocardial Infarction

Suspicion of AMI?

Yes

Prehospital Setting:

Primary Treatment::

- ABCs
- **Oxygen**
- Start IV
- ECG, vital signs
- **Nitroglycerin**
- Pain relief with narcotics

Optional treatment:

- Screening for thrombolytic therapy
- 12-lead ECG, computer analysis, transmission to emergency department
- Initiation of thrombolytic therapy

Hospital Setting

Assessment

- ABCs
- Vital signs with automatic BP, pulse oximeter
- **Oxygen** at 4 L/min 🕮 87
- Start IV
- 12-lead ECG (reviewed by M.D.)
- Brief, targeted history and physical
- Determine eligibility for thrombolytic therapy
- Chest roentgenogram
- Blood studies (electrolytes, enzymes, coagulation studies)
- Consult as needed

If there is evidence of coronary thrombosis, consider some of the following treatments

Treatment:

- **Nitroglycerin** SL, paste or spray (if the systolic BP is >90 mmHg)
- **Morphine**, IV
- **Aspirin**, PO
- **Thrombolytic agents**
- **Nitroglycerin**, IV 🕮 84
- **β-Blockers**, IV
- **Heparin**, IV
- Percutaneous transluminal coronary angioplasty

Section 5

ACLS Medications

Special Information

- dosages are **bolded** for easy visualization.
- indications are listed in larger size lettering for easy visualization.
- references to other critical information are identified by the "🕮" **symbol** followed by a page number.

Adenosine

Dosage:

- **6 mg, rapid IV push** (1-3 seconds).

If, after 1-2 min, cardioversion does not occur, administer:

- **12 mg, rapid IV push** (1-3 seconds). May be repeated once if necessary.

Indications:

- Paroxysmal supraventricular tachycardia (PSVT) (Class I) 📖 64.
- Wide-complex tachycardia of uncertain type (Class IIa) 📖 64.

Used to: Suppress supraventricular tachycardia.

Actions: Depresses AV and sinus node activity.

Side Effects:

CVS Transient bradycardia and ventricular ectopy are common after termination of PSVT with adenosine.

CNS Dizziness, headache.

Others Facial flushing, shortness of breath, chest pain, and nausea.

Precautions:

Should not be used in:
Second- or third-degree heart block.
Sick sinus syndrome.
Known hypersensitivity to the drug.
Use with caution in: asthma patients.

Additional Information

Because adenosine produces a short-lived response of less than 5 seconds, PSVT may reoccur. Side effects usually resolve spontaneously within 1-2 minutes. Administer adenosine directly into a vein or administration port closest to the patient. Flush the line with IV solution after administering the drug.

Atropine Sulfate

Dosage:

In symptomatic bradycardia:

- **0.5-1.0 mg** (repeated q. 3-5 min, to a total of 3 mg or 0.04 mg/kg).

In asystole/PEA:

- **1 mg** (may be repeated in 3-5 min, to a total of 0.04 mg/kg).

Indications:

- Symptomatic bradycardia (Class I).
- Bradycardia with PVCs 🕮 63.
- Asystole (Class IIa) 🕮 62.
- PEA (with rate <60 or relative bradycardia) 🕮 62.

Used to:

Increase the heart rate.

Actions:

Blocks parasympathetic nervous system, enhancing both SA node automaticity and AV conduction. Allows heart to return to its inherent rate or sympathetic nervous system to increase heart rate.

Side Effects:

CVS Tachycardia, palpitations, angina, PVCs, VF/VT, hypotension.

CNS Headache, dizziness, anxiety, blurred vision, dilated pupils, ataxia.

Others Dry mouth/nose, difficulty swallowing, N/V, difficulty urinating, flushed, hot skin, **may exacerbate ischemia**.

Precautions:

Should not be used in: Tachycardia, atrial flutter/fibrillation, glaucoma.
Use with caution in: Type II or 3rd-degree (wide-complex) AV block (Class III), AMI.

In symptomatic patients, don't wait for IV access or atropine to take effect before employing TCP.

Additional Information

- Shorter dosing intervals may be helpful in severe clinical conditions.
- May be administered endotracheally at 2 to 2.5 times IV dose.

Bretylium Tosylate

Dosage:

<u>In ventricular fibrillation</u>:

- **5 mg/kg**, rapid IV push (repeat q. 5 min at 10 mg/kg to a maximum dose of 30-35 mg/kg).

<u>In ventricular tachycardia with a pulse</u>:

- **5-10 mg/kg**, over 8-10 min.

Indications:

<u>Refractory ventricular ectopy (Class IIb)</u>:

- Wide-complex tachycardia 📖 64.
- Ventricular tachycardia 📖 64.
- Ventricular fibrillation 📖 60.

Used to:

Suppress ventricular dysrhythmias and raise the fibrillation threshold.

Actions:

Initial sympathomimetic effects (<20 min) followed by blockade (within 1 to 2 hours) of norepinephrine release from peripheral sympathetic nerves.

Side Effects:

CVS	Possible transient increase in blood pressure or heart rate, hypotension, bradycardia.
CNS	Dizziness, vertigo, syncope.
Others	N/V, angina, nasal stuffiness.

Precautions:

<u>Should not be used in</u>: known aortic stenosis, torsades de pointes.
<u>Use with extreme caution in</u>: arrhythmias due to digitalis toxicity.

Additional Information

<u>If the rhythm is successfully converted administer</u>:

- a bretylium **infusion of 1-2 mg/min**.

Calcium Chloride

Dosage:

- **2-4 mg/kg (10% solution) slow IV push**. May be repeated at ten min intervals as considered necessary.

Indications:

Class IIa for:

- Acute hyperkalemia (elevated potassium).
- Acute hypocalcemia (decreased calcium).
- Overdose of a calcium channel blocker (nifedipine, verapamil, etc.) 📖 90.

Used to:

Replace electrolytes.

Actions:

Increases myocardial contractility.

Side Effects:

CVS Arrhythmias (bradycardia, asystole, VF), hypotension, may cause coronary and cerebral vasospasm.

Others Chalky or metallic taste.

Precautions:

Should not be used in:
Patients receiving digitalis.
Extravasation may cause tissue necrosis.

Additional Information

- IV line should be flushed between calcium chloride and sodium bicarbonate administration.

Diazepam

Dosage:

- **5-10 mg, slow IV push** (q. 5 min, up to a maximum of 20 mg).

Indications:

- Premedication prior to cardioversion 📖 18, 64.
- Acute anxiety states.

Used to: Sedate patients.

Actions: Depresses the central nervous system, produces a transient amnesia.

Side Effects:

CVS	Hypotension, reflex tachycardia.
CNS	Respiratory depression, apnea, drowsiness, ataxia, transient amnesia.
Others	Warmth, pain, burning or phlebitis extending from IV site; may cause thrombosis, N/V.

Precautions:

Should not be used in:
Patients with a history of hypersensitivity to the drug.
Respiratory depression.
Hypotension.

Additional Information

- Has short duration of effect.
- Some recommend including an analgesic along with the administration of the sedative that precedes cardioversion.
- Is also used in treatment of seizures.

Diltiazem

Dosage:

- **0.25 mg/kg, IV push,** followed by a second dose of **0.35 mg/kg.**
- May also be used as a maintenance **infusion of 5-15 mg/h** to control the ventricular rate in atrial fibrillation.

Indications:

- Atrial fibrillation/flutter 🕮 64.
- Refractory atrial tachycardia with normal or elevated BP.

Used to:

Suppress supraventricular tachycardia.

Actions:

Blocks entry of calcium into cells, slowing conduction and increasing refractoriness in the AV node. Diltiazem may terminate reentrant arrhythmias that require AV conduction for their continuation.

Side Effects:

CVS	Conduction disturbances, arrhythmia, hypotension, bradycardia, CHF, peripheral edema.
CNS	Headache, fatigue, drowsiness, dizziness, nervousness, CNS depression, confusion, insomnia.
Others	N/V, flushing, rash.

Precautions:

May decrease myocardial contractility and exacerbate congestive heart failure in patients with severe left ventricular dysfunction.

Dobutamine

Dosage:

- **2-20 mcg/kg/min, IV infusion.**

Indications:

Decreased cardiac output:

- Depressed myocardial function (when the systolic BP is >100 mm Hg and diastolic BP is normotensive) 📖 66.
- Cardiogenic shock, CHF 📖 67.

Used to:

Increase cardiac output by increasing myocardial contractility.

Actions:

Strong β_1 stimulant (increased contractility) that has little effect on the heart rate. Also has a slight β_2 stimulatory effect (some vasodilation).

Side Effects:

CVS Palpitations, PVCs, tachycardia, angina, increased BP.

CNS Headache, tremor.

Others N/V.

Precautions:

Should not be used in:
Hypovolemia.
Uncorrected tachycardia.
Signs of myocardial ischemia.

Dobutamine should not be used alone in the seriously ill patient with systolic BP > about 100 mm Hg.

Additional Information

- β-blockers may inhibit effects.
- Alkaline solutions may inactivate.
- Sometimes used with Dopamine or Nitroprusside.
- Less adverse cardiac effects than Dopamine.

Dopamine

Dosage:

- **2-20 mcg/kg/min, IV infusion,** titrated to effect (add Norepinephrine if Dopamine is >20 mcg/kg/min).

Indications:

Depressed cardiac function:

- Cardiogenic shock (when the systolic BP is 70-100 mm Hg).
- Other shock (hemodynamically significant hypotension) 📖 66.
- Refractory bradycardia 📖 63.

Used to:

Increase cardiac output and BP.

Actions:

Dopaminergic stimulant (dilates renal and mesenteric blood vessels) at doses of 1-2 mcg/kg/min, β_1 stimulant (increases cardiac output) at 2-10 mcg/kg/min, α stimulant (peripheral vasoconstriction and increased pulmonary occlusive pressure) at <10 mcg/kg/min.

Side Effects:

CVS Tachycardia, ectopy, palpitations, angina.

CNS Headache, tremor.

Others N/V, dyspnea, tissue necrosis, warmth, pain, burning extending from IV site.

Precautions:

Should not be used in:

Hypotension caused by hypovolemia.
Uncorrected tachyarrhythmias.
Ventricular fibrillation.
Pheochromocytoma.

Monoamine oxidase inhibitors potentiate the effects of dopamine.

Additional Information

- If norepinephrine is used to increase the BP, move to Dopamine and stop Norepinephrine when the BP improves.

Epinephrine (1:10,000)

Dosage:

<u>In cardiac arrest</u>:

- **1.0 mg, IV push** (may be repeated every 3-5 min).

<u>In refractory bradycardia:</u>

- **2-20 mcg/min, IV infusion**.

Indications:

- Ventricular fibrillation/pulseless ventricular tachycardia 🕮 60.
- Asystole 🕮 62.
- Pulseless electrical activity 🕮 62.
- Refractory bradycardia 🕮 63.

Used to:

Increase cardiac output.

Actions:

Strong α and β stimulant (increased HR, BP). Its α adrenergic effects increase myocardial and cerebral blood flow during CPR.

Side Effects:

CVS Palpitations, tachycardia, angina, ectopic beats, palpitations, increased BP.

CNS Nervousness, anxiety, headache, tremor, pupil dilation.

Additional Information

- May be administered via ET route at 2 to 2.5 times the IV dose.
- If unsuccessful at recommended dose, higher doses can be considered:
  - **<u>intermediate</u>: 2-5 mg IV push,** q. 3-5 min.
  - **<u>escalating</u>: 1 mg-3 mg-5 mg IV push** (3 min apart).
  - **<u>high</u>: 0.1 mg/kg IV push,** q. 3-5 min
- Follow each dose of epinephrine (given by peripheral injection) with a 20-ml flush of IV fluid to ensure effective distribution of the drug into the central compartment.

Furosemide

Dosage:

- **0.5-1.0 mg/kg, IV push** (typically 20-80 mg).

Indications:

Circulatory overload:

- Acute pulmonary edema 🕮 66.
- Congestive heart failure 🕮 66.
- Hypertensive crisis.
- Cerebral edema after cardiac arrest.

Used to:

Increase urine output and dilate blood vessels.

Actions:

Inhibits reabsorption of sodium and chloride in the proximal and distal renal tubule and loop of Henle. This action results in the excretion of more sodium and water. Also has a direct venodilating effect.

Side Effects:

CVS	Potassium depletion with attendant dysrhythmias, hyperglycemia.
CNS	Vertigo, visual/auditory disturbances.
Others	N/V, dehydration.

Precautions:

Should not be used in:

Pregnant women.
Hypokalemia.
Patients who are allergic to sulfas or thiazides.
Hypovolemia.

Isoproterenol

Dosage:

2-10 mcg/min, IV infusion (titrated to a heart rate of 60 per min).

Indications:

- Hemodynamically compromising bradycardia refractory to atropine.
- Hemodynamically significant bradycardia in denervated hearts of heart transplant patients (Class IIa) 📖 63.
- Refractory torsades de pointes (Class IIa).

Used to:

Increase the heart rate.

Actions:

β_1 and β_2 stimulant with potent inotropic and chronotropic properties that increase cardiac output and myocardial work.

Side Effects:

CVS Hypotension, palpitations, angina, may lead to worsening of ischemia/infarction.

CNS Dizziness, anxiety, nervousness, headache, tremors.

Others Flushing, sweating, dyspnea, N/V.

Precautions:

Should not be used in:
Patients with cardiac arrest, hypotension, or ischemic heart disease.
Preexistent tachycardias, PEA, asystole.
Digitalis toxicity or hypokalemia.
Hepatic or renal insufficiency.

Do not mix with epinephrine.

Additional Information

- **Isoproterenol should be used with extreme caution, if used at all**. At low doses it is Class IIb (possibly helpful); at higher doses it is Class III (harmful).

Lidocaine

Dosage:

If hemodynamically stable:

- **1-1.5 mg/kg, IV push** (repeated q. 5-10 min, at 0.5-0.75 mg/kg, if necessary, to a total of 3 mg/kg).

In ventricular fibrillation/tachycardia:

- **1.5 mg/kg, IV push** (repeat q. 3-5 min to a loading dose of 3 mg/kg).

Indications:

Ventricular ectopy:

- PVCs.
- Ventricular tachycardia 📖 64.
- Wide-complex tachycardia 📖 64.
- Refractory ventricular fibrillation 📖 60.

Used to:

Suppress ventricular dysrhythmias, raise fibrillation threshold.

Actions:

Reduces velocity of electrical impulses through conduction system and disparity in action potential duration between ischemic and normal myocardial zones.

Side Effects:

CVS Hypotension, bradycardia, conduction disturbances.

CNS CNS depression, drowsiness, dizziness, respiratory depression, numbness/tingling, slurred speech, confusion, tremor, seizures.

Precautions:

Should not be used in:
3rd-degree AV block (with ventricular escape).
Bradycardia-related PVCs.
Idioventricular rhythm.
Give lidocaine at half the initial dose in: decreased cardiac output (e.g., acute MI, CHF, shock), patients older than 70 years, and those with hepatic dysfunction.

Additional Information

- May be administered via ET route at 2 to 2.5 times IV dose.
- In stable conditions, the IV bolus of lidocaine is followed by a **2-4 mg/min, IV infusion**.

Magnesium Sulfate

Dosage:

In recurrent or refractory VF/VT:

- **1-2 gm**, diluted in 100 ml of D_5W, **administered IV push over 1-2 min**.

In documented hypomagnesemia:

- **1-2 gm,** diluted in 50-100 ml of D_5W, **administered over 5-60 min**. An infusion of 0.5-1.0 grams/hour should follow for up to 24 hours.

Indications:

- Torsades de pointes.
- Suspected hypomagnesium state.
- Severe recurrent or refractory ventricular fibrillation 📖 61.

Used to:

Reverse refractory ventricular fibrillation, hypomagnesemia.

Actions:

Stabilizes muscle cell membranes by interacting with the sodium/potassium exchange.

Side Effects:

CVS Cardiac arrest.
CNS Drowsiness, respiratory depression.

Precautions:

Should not be used in:
Renal disease.
Heart block.

Caution should be used when magnesium is administered to safeguard against clinically significant hypotension or asystole.

Morphine Sulfate

Dosage:

- **1-3 mg, slow IV push** (as often as q. 5 min).

Indications:

- Pulmonary edema due to CHF (Class IIb) 📖 67.
- Pain associated with AMI 📖 68.

Used to:

Relieve pain and dilate blood vessels.

Actions:

Analgesia, vasodilation (which reduces myocardial oxygen consumption), and sedation.

Side Effects:

CVS Hypotension, bradycardia.

CNS Respiratory depression/apnea, CNS depression, euphoria, drowsiness, dizziness, weakness, paradoxical CNS stimulation, nervousness, anxiety, headache, seizure, coma.

Others Flushing, N/V, pupil constriction.

Precautions:

Should not be used in:
Head injury.
Volume depletion.
Undiagnosed abdominal pain.
Patients with hypersensitivity to the drug.

Naloxone should be available to reverse significant side effects such as respiratory depression or hypotension.

Nitroglycerin

Dosage:

With chest pain:

- **0.3 to 0.6 mg, tablet SL** (may be repeated q. 3-5 min up to a total of 1.2 mg).
- Can also be administered as a spray.

In congestive heart failure:

- **10-20 mcg/min, IV infusion**.

Indications:

- Ischemic chest pain 📖 66.
- AMI 📖 68.
- Selected cases of pulmonary edema due to CHF 📖 68.

Used to:

Improve coronary circulation and reduce myocardial workload.

Actions:

Smooth muscle relaxant, reduces cardiac workload, dilates coronary arteries, dilates systemic arteries.

Side Effects:

CVS	Hypotension, bradycardia, paradoxical angina, reflex tachycardia, palpitations.
CNS	Throbbing headache, dizziness, weakness.
Others	Flushing, feelings of warmth, N/V, hypoxemia caused by increased pulmonary ventilation-perfusion mismatch, methemoglobinemia.

Precautions:

Should not be used in:

Increased intracranial pressure.
Hypotension.
Glaucoma.
Hypovolemia.
Suspected tamponade or pericarditis.

Nitroprusside

Dosage:

- **0.1-5.0 mcg/kg/min, IV infusion.**

Indications:

- Acute hypertensive crisis 🕮 66.
- CHF, cardiogenic shock 🕮 67.

Used to:

Improve cardiac output.

Actions:

Potent, rapid-acting direct peripheral vasodilator used to treat heart failure and hypertension. Nitroprusside reduces peripheral arterial resistance (afterload).

Side Effects:

CVS Hypotension, reflex tachycardia, palpitations, angina.

CNS CNS depression.

Others Thiocyanate toxicity, may cause warmth, pain, burning or phlebitis extending from IV site.

Precautions:

<u>Should not be used in</u>:
Compensatory hypertension.
Dissecting aneurysm.

Reduce the BP slowly.
Extravasation causes tissue necrosis.

Norepinephrine

Dosage:

- **0.5-1 mcg/min, IV infusion titrated to effect up to 30 mcg/minute.**

Indications:

Hypotension:

- Severe inappropriate systemic vascular resistance (when the systolic BP is <70 mm Hg) 🕮 66.

Used to:

Increase cardiac output, arterial pressure.

Actions:

Strong α stimulant with some β stimulating properties.

Side Effects:

CVS	Tachycardia, hypertension.
CNS	Anxiety, severe headaches.
Others	Tissue necrosis, N/V, sweating.

Precautions:

Should not be used in:
Hypotension resulting from hypovolemia.
Hypoxia, hypercarbia.

Use with extreme caution in AMI.

Oxygen

Dosage:

<u>In hypoxia</u>:

- Patients in critical condition should receive **100%**.

<u>In acute myocardial infarction</u>:

- **4-6 liters** per min.

<u>In cardiac arrest</u>:

- **100%** should always be used.

Indications:

- Prevention or treatment of hypoxemia (global or local) from any cause.
- Myocardial ischemia/infarction.
- Respiratory difficulty.
- Cardiac arrest.

Used to:

Relieve hypoxemia.

Actions:

Increases PaO_2 and hemoglobin oxygen saturation.

Side Effects:

None with short-term use.

Precautions:

A concentration of 24%-35% oxygen should be used when the stable patient has a history of COPD.

Procainamide

Dosage:

<u>Ventricular tachycardia</u>:

- **20-30 mg/min, IV push**.

<u>Refractory ventricular fibrillation</u>:

- **30 mg/min, IV push**.

Indications:

<u>Refractory</u>:

- Frequent PVCs.
- Ventricular fibrillation/tachycardia 🕮 61.
- Wide-complex tachycardia 🕮 64.

Used to:

Suppress ventricular ectopy and raise the fibrillation threshold.

Actions:

Slows conduction through myocardium by increasing electrical threshold of ventricle, His-Purkinje system.

Side Effects:

CVS	Hypotension, reflex tachycardia, ventricular fibrillation, AV block, widened QRS, bradycardia, asystole.
CNS	CNS depression, hallucination, confusion, dizziness, seizures.
Others	N/V, fever.

Precautions:

<u>Should not be used in</u>:

Complete AV block, bradycardia.

Digitalis toxicity.

Preexisting QT prolongation.

Torsades de pointes.

Additional Information

- End points of procainamide administration are: suppression of the dysrhythmia, total of 17 mg/kg given, more than 50% widening of QRS complex, or hypotension ensues.
- If procainamide suppresses VT, start a continuous infusion at 1-4 mg/min. The maintenance dose should be reduced in renal failure.

Sodium Bicarbonate

Dosage:
- **1 mEq/kg, IV push.**

Indications:
Refractory cardiac arrest:
- Known preexisting hyperkalemia (Class I).
- Known preexisting bicarbonate-responsive acidosis.
- Overdose with tricyclic antidepressants (Class IIa).
- To alkalize the urine in drug overdose (Class IIa).
- If intubated and continued long arrest interval (Class IIb).
- Upon return of spontaneous circulation following long arrest interval (Class IIb).

Used to: Reverse metabolic acidosis.

Actions: Buffers metabolic acids.

Side Effects:
CVS Increased vascular volume.
Others Lowers serum potassium, buildup of CO_2.

Precautions:
Should not be used in:
Hypokalemia.
CHF.
Hypoxic lactic acidosis such as that which occurs in nonintubated patients with prolonged CPR.

Verapamil

Dosage:

- **2.5 to 5 mg, slow IV push** (over 2 min).

If tachycardia is not resolved in 15-30 min:

- **5-10 mg, slow IV push** (repeated q. 15-30 min to a maximum of 20 mg).

Indications:

Refractory supraventricular tachycardia:

- Narrow complex PSVT refractory to vagal maneuver and adenosine with normal/elevated BP 📖 65.
- Rate control in atrial fibrillation.
- Ventricular rate control in atrial flutter, multifocal atrial tachycardia.

Used to:

Suppress supraventricular tachyarrhythmias.

Actions:

Calcium channel blocker, antiarrhythmic.

Side Effects:

CVS Hypotension, AV or sinus blocks, bradycardia, asystole, tachycardia, may exacerbate CHF/pulmonary edema.

CNS Dizziness, headache, seizures.

Others Nausea, abdominal discomfort, sweaty, flushing.

Precautions:

Should not be used in:
Severe hypotension, cardiogenic shock, severe CHF, sinus bradycardia, 2nd- or 3rd-degree AV block, sick sinus. Patients receiving intravenous beta adrenergic blocking drugs.

May decrease myocardial contractility and exacerbate congestive heart failure in patients with left ventricular dysfunction.

Additional Information

Given only in dysrhythmias known with certainty to be supraventricular.

Medication Calculations

Use the formulas below to calculate IV solution drip rates per minute, the number of ml needed to deliver IV push medications, and the drip rates per minute needed to deliver medications via IV infusion.

Formula for figuring IV volumes to be administered over a given time:

$$\text{gtt/min} = \frac{\text{volume to be infused} \times \text{gtt/ml of administration set}}{\text{total time of infusion in minutes}}$$

e.g. You are instructed to administer 35 ml of IV fluid over 40 minutes using a microdrip administration set. *Your formula is: 35 ml × 60 gtt/ml = 2,100 gtt divided by 40 minutes = 52.5 gtt/minute (rounded to 50 gtt/minute) you need to administer.*

Formula for figuring volumes to be administered for IV push medications:

$$\text{volume administered } (x) = \frac{\text{volume on hand} \times \text{desired dosage}}{\text{concentration on hand}}$$

e.g. You are instructed to administer 5 mg of diazepam to premedicate your tachycardic patient prior to synchronized cardioversion. Your kit is supplied with 2 ml prefilled syringes containing 10 mg of diazepam. *Your formula is: 2 ml × 5 mg = 10 ml/mg divided by 10 mg = 1 ml (the amount you are to administer).*

Formula for figuring volumes to be administered for weight-dependent IV push medications:

Step 1: DIVIDE the patient's weight (in pounds) by 2.2 to reveal the patient's weight in kilograms.
Step 2: MULTIPLY the weight in kilograms by the prescribed dose.
Step 3: Use the formula below to determine the number of ml needed to deliver the desired dose.

$$\text{volume administered } (x) = \frac{\text{volume on hand} \times \text{desired dosage}}{\text{concentration on hand}}$$

e.g. You are instructed to administer 1 mg/kg of lidocaine to your 135 pound patient who is displaying multifocal PVCs. Your kit has 5 ml prefilled syringes containing 100 mg of lidocaine. Your formula is as follows: *135 pounds divided by 2.2 = 61.36 (rounded off to 60) kg. 1 mg × 60 kg = 60 mg. 5 ml × 60 mg = 300 ml/mg divided by 100 mg = 3 ml (the amount you will administer).*

Formula for figuring drop (gtt) rate for medications delivered via IV infusion:

$$\text{gtt/min} = \frac{\text{volume on hand} \times \text{desired dosage}}{\text{concentration on hand}} \times \text{gtt of administration set}$$

e.g. You are instructed to administer lidocaine at 2 mg per minute IV infusion to your 135 pound patient who is displaying multifocal PVCs. Your kit includes 10 ml prefilled syringes that each contain 1 gm of lidocaine. Your protocol calls for you to mix it in 250 ml of normal saline and use a microdrip administration set to deliver it. *Your formula is as follows: 250 ml × 2 mg/min = 500 ml/mg/min divided by 1,000 mg = 0.5 ml/min × 60 gtts/ml = 30 gtts/min.*